Essentials of Pharmacology
for Health Occupations

Essentials of Pharmacology for Health Occupations

RUTH WOODROW, R. N., M. A.

Instructor, Pharmacology
Coordinator, Continuing Education
Sarasota County Vocational-Technical Center
Sarasota, Florida

A WILEY MEDICAL PUBLICATION

JOHN WILEY & SONS

New York • Chichester • Brisbane • Toronto • Singapore

The following figures are reprinted with permission from B. W. Narrow and K. B. Buschle, *Fundamentals of Nursing Practice,* © 1982, John Wiley & Sons, Inc.: Figures 4.4, 4.5, 4.6, 4.13, 9.6, 9.7, 9.8, 9.9, 9.10, 9.12, 9.13, 9.14, 9.15, 9.19, 9.20, 9.21, 9.24, and 23.1.

The following tables are reprinted with permission from T. R. Lankford and P. M. Jacobs-Steward, *Foundations of Normal and Therapeutic Nutrition,* © 1986, John Wiley & Sons, Inc.: Tables 11.1 and 11.2.

The following photos were produced by Chuck Kennedy, photographer, The Chuck Kennedy Group, Inc., Sarasota, Florida: Figures 1.1, 3.2, 4.2, 4.7, 4.8, 4.9, 4.10, 4.11, 4.12, 5.2, 8.1, 8.2, 8.3, 8.4, 8.5, 8.6, 9.1, 9.3, 9.4, 9.5, 14.1, 14.2, and 23.2.

The following figures were drawn by Masako Herman: Figures 2.1, 3.3, 3.4, 4.1, 4.3, 7.1, 8.7, 8.8, 8.10, 8.11, 9.16, 9.17, 9.18, 9.22, and 9.23.

The following figures were drawn by Judy Avery, Commercial Art Department, Sarasota County Vocational-Technical Center, Sarasota, Florida: Figures 3.1, 18.1, and 20.1.

The author and publisher have made a conscientious effort to ensure that the drug information in this book is accurate and in accord with accepted standards at the time of publication. However, pharmacology is a rapidly changing science, so readers are advised, before administering any drug, to check the package insert provided by the manufacturer for the recommended dose, for contraindications for administration, and for added warnings and precautions. This recommendation is especially important for new, infrequently used, or highly toxic drugs.

Library of Congress Cataloging in Publication Data:

Woodrow, Ruth.
    Essentials of pharmacology for health occupations.

    (A Wiley medical publication)
    Includes index.
    1. Pharmacology. 2. Drugs. 3. Pharmacology — Examinations, questions, etc. 4. Drugs — Examinations, questions, etc. I. Title. II. Series. [DNLM: 1. Drug Therapy. 2. Pharmacology.   QV 4 W893e]

RM300.W67   1987   615.5'8   86-32451
ISBN 0-471-84542-6 (pbk.)

Printed in the United States of America

10   9   8   7   6   5   4   3   2

To my students,
who inspired me by their need,
encouraged me with their questions and comments,
and rewarded me with their success.

Contributor

Karen DeHahn, B. S. N.
Instructor, Practical Nursing Program
Sarasota County Vocational-Technical Center
Sarasota, Florida

Consultants

Phyllis Eastwood, R. N., R. E. M. T., M.Ed.
Department Chairman/Instructor, EMT/Paramedic Program
Sarasota County Vocational-Technical Center
Sarasota, Florida

Edward A. Kalchbrenner, R. Ph.
Director of Pharmacy
Venice Hospital
Venice, Florida

Harriette Laronge, C. M. A.
Instructor, Medical Assisting Program
Sarasota County Vocational-Technical Center
Sarasota, Florida

Margaret Schettler, R. N.
Instructor, Practical Nursing Program
Sarasota County Vocational-Technical Center
Sarasota, Florida

Miriam Smith, M. S., R. D.
Consultant Dietitian
Venice Hospital
Venice, Florida

Leo Wojcechowskyj, R. Ph.
Director of Pharmacy Services
Sarasota Palms Hospital
Sarasota, Florida

Preface

This book is designed as:

- A basic text for nursing students, medical assistant students, and students of other allied health occupations
- A continuing education update for practitioners in the health field
- Part of a refresher program for practitioners returning to health occupations
- A supplemental or reference book for practitioners wishing to extend their knowledge beyond basic training in specific health occupations

The purpose of this book is to provide an extensive framework of knowledge that can be acquired within a limited time frame. It will be especially helpful to students in 1-year training programs with limited time allotted to the study of medications. For those in longer programs, it can be used as the basis for more extensive study. It is appropriate as a required text in training those who will administer medications. It has been especially designed to meet the needs of students in nursing and medical assistant programs. However, students in allied health programs will find the concise format adaptable to their needs also.

This text has been field-tested in several classes with students in various health occupations. Students who have already used this book for updating or supplemental education include registered nurses, licensed practical nurses, medical assistants, and paramedics.

Those employed in health occupations now have increased responsibilities for providing the necessary information to patients regarding the safe administration of medications, side effects, and interactions. The quantity of information could be overwhelming and confusing unless presented in a comprehensive and concise manner.

The organization of the text in a concise format eliminates unnecessary detail that may tend to overwhelm or confuse the student. Outdated or infrequently used medications, obsolete information, and complex descriptions are eliminated. The information presented is both factual and functional.

Part I carefully introduces the student to the fascinating subject of drugs, their sources, and uses. Calculations are simplified into two optional, step-by-step processes. Review questions at the end of each chapter help the student master the information. Administration checklists allow the student to put the information into practice. Illustrations facilitate the learning process.

Part II organizes the drugs according to the body systems. Each classification is described, along with characteristics of typical drugs, side effects, cautions, interactions, and patient education for each category. A worksheet at the end of each chapter helps the student organize the information into outline form. A comprehensive review quiz follows both Part I and Part II.

To the Student Studying Pharmacology

Other students, such as you, have helped me put this book together. They have learned that the study of medications can be a fascinating one. They tell me that this book has helped them to develop confidence and competence in dispensing medications and information about drugs to their patients. You will find this is only the beginning, a framework upon which you will build a vast store of useful knowledge.

Students have told me that the objectives, review questions, and worksheets were tremendously helpful to them. Organization is the key to acquiring large quantities of information. You will be amazed at all you have learned when you complete this book.

Keep growing and learning and questioning all of your life.

RUTH WOODROW

Contents

List of Tables

Essentials of Pharmacology
for Health Occupations

PART I

Introduction

1

Consumer Safety

OBJECTIVES

Upon completion of this chapter, the student will be able to:

1. Explain what is meant by drug standards.
2. Name the first drug law passed in this country for consumer safety, and give the year it was passed.
3. Summarize the provisions of the Federal Food, Drug, and Cosmetic Act of 1938, and identify the government agency that enforces the act.
4. Interpret what is meant by *USP/NF.*
5. Summarize the provisions of the Controlled Substances Act of 1970.
6. Explain what is meant by a DEA number.
7. Define schedules of controlled substances, and differentiate between C-I to C-V schedules.
8. State several responsibilities you have in the dispensing of medications, as a direct result of the three major drug laws described in this chapter.

Your decision to pursue a career in the health field probably took a great deal of thought. No doubt you have questioned whether you will be able to handle the unique situations that arise in a clinic, health care facility, or physician's office. Have you ever stopped to consider the impact *you* will make on the lives of others as a health care worker? Not only can you make a tremendous difference in the efficiency of the office's patient flow, but you can have a positive impact on your friends and family, as well as the patient.

It is inevitable that you will receive phone calls and questions about medications, prescriptions, and drug therapy. A great majority of patients are far too inhibited to tell their physician that they do not understand about their medications. They feel much more at ease discussing their questions with the health care worker. Your potential for informing others with knowledgeable answers about medications can be quite an asset!

The key to reaching that potential is having knowledgeable answers. A serious, responsible attitude about all aspects of drug therapy is imperative. Consider yourself a potential prime resource of medication information for your friends, family, and future patients, as you begin to examine the foundations of facts about drugs. It may be necessary for you to clarify some of the layperson's misunderstandings about the legalities of dispensing medications. Consider the following misconceptions and facts.

FALLACY	FACT
Only nurses can give medications to patients.	Trained and certified health care workers who may legally give medications include physicians, paramedics, medical office assistants, and practical and registered nurses.
Only physicians may write prescriptions.	Dentists, physicians, veterinarians, nurse practitioners, and registered pharmacists may write prescriptions for their specific field of work, within limitations. For example, veterinarians write prescriptions for animal use only.
Prescriptions are required for narcotics only.	Specific drugs ruled illegal to purchase without the use of a prescription include: • Those that need to be controlled because they are addictive and tend to be abused and dangerous (e.g., depressants, stimulants, psychedelics, and narcotics). • Those that may cause dangerous health threats from side effects if taken incorrectly (e.g., antibiotics, cardiac drugs, tranquilizers, etc.).
All drugs produced in the U.S. are made in federally approved laboratories.	Numerous undercover, illegal laboratories exist and operate within the U.S. today.

Drug Laws

The matter of dispensing drugs in the United States is specifically addressed by laws passed in the 1900s. Scientific advances, progress, and changes in society in the last century have made it necessary for drug laws to be set for our safety. Although substances have been taken into the body for their effects for centuries, so many are being produced today that *consumer safety* is now a critical issue.

Drug standards are rules set to assure consumers that they get what they pay for. The law says that all preparations called by the same drug name must be of *uniform strength, quality, and purity.*

Because of drug standardization, when you take a prescription to be filled, you are assured of getting the same basic drug, in the same amount and quality, no matter to which pharmacy or to which part of the country you take the prescription to be filled. According to drug standards, the drug companies must not add other active ingredients or varying amounts of chemicals to a specific drug preparation. They must meet the drug standards (federally approved requirements) for the specified strength, quality, and purity of the drug.

Unlike our predecessors, we no longer have to wonder what ingredients, if any (other than sugar and water, or alcohol), are in the "medicinal waters" being sold.

In the market of illegal (illicit) drugs, the lack of enforcement of drug standards is the consumer's danger. With no controls on the quality of illegal drugs (because they are unapproved for safety), many deaths have occurred from overdose. Consider the heroin user, accustomed to very poor quality heroin, who accidently overdoses when given a much higher quality of heroin from a new source.

The laws that have evolved to provide consumer safety can be summed up by three major acts. They are described in the order in which they became necessary for consumer safety.

1906 PURE FOOD AND DRUG ACT

First government attempt to establish consumer protection in the manufacture of drugs and foods.

Required all drugs marketed in the U.S. to meet *minimal* standards of strength, purity, and quality.

Demanded that drug preparations containing morphine have a labeled container indicating the ingredient morphine.

Established two references of *officially* approved drugs. Before 1906, information about drugs was handed down from generation to generation. No official written resources existed. After the 1906 legislation, two references specified the official U.S. standards for making each drug. Those references, listed below, have since been combined into one book, referred to as the *USP/NF:*

• *United States Pharmacopoeia (USP)*

• *National Formulary (NF)*

1938 FEDERAL FOOD, DRUG, AND COSMETIC ACT AND AMENDMENTS OF 1951 AND 1965

Established the Food and Drug Administration (FDA) under the Department of Health and Welfare to enforce the provisions of the act.

Established *more specific* regulations to prevent adulteration of (tampering with) drugs, foods, and cosmetics:

- All labels must be accurate and must include generic names.
- All new products must be approved by the FDA before public release.
- "Warning" labels must be present on certain preparations for example, "May cause drowsiness," "may cause nervousness," and "may be habit-forming."
- Certain drugs must be labeled with the legend (inscription): "Caution — federal law prohibits dispensing without a prescription." Thus, the term *legend drugs* refers to such preparations. The act also designated which drugs can be sold without a prescription.
- Prescription and nonprescription drugs must be shown to be *effective* as well as *safe*.

The importance of the timing of this law should be noted. It came about as the answer to a disastrous occurrence in 1937. A sulfa preparation, not adequately tested for safety, was responsible for 100 deaths that year. Thus the need was recognized for more proof of the safety and effectiveness of new drugs.

1970 CONTROLLED SUBSTANCES ACT

Established the Drug Enforcement Administration (DEA) as a bureau of the Department of Justice to enforce the provisions of the act.

Set much tighter controls on a specific group of drugs: those that were being abused by society; the name of the act indicates that such *substances needed to be controlled*. They include depressants, stimulants, psychedelics, and narcotics. The act:

- Isolated the abused and addicting drugs into five levels, or schedules, according to their degree of danger: C-I, C-II, C-III, C-IV, or C-V.
- Demanded security of controlled substances; anyone (e.g., pharmacists, hospitals, physicians, and drug companies) who dispenses, receives, sells, or destroys controlled substances must keep on hand special DEA forms, indicating the exact current inventory, and a 2-year inventory of every controlled substance transaction.
- Set limitations on the use of prescriptions; guidelines were established for each of the five schedules of controlled substances, regulating the number of times a drug may be prescribed in a 6-month period as well as for which schedules prescriptions may be phoned in to the pharmacy, and so on.
- Demanded that each prescriber of theses substances register with the DEA and obtain a DEA registration number, to be present on their prescriptions of controlled substances; drug manufacturers must also be registered and identified with their own DEA numbers, as must pharmacists, physicians, veterinarians, and so on.

The five schedules of controlled substances are arranged with the potentially most dangerous at level I and the least dangerous at level V. The higher the level, the stricter the restrictions for control by the DEA. Thus, level I is the strictest.

Drugs are frequently added, deleted, or moved from one schedule to another. If, for example, the DEA determines that drug A is becoming more of a societal problem, with an increased incidence of overdoses, drug A may be moved from the C-IV schedule to C-III. It is extremely important that the health care worker keep informed of any changes in drug scheduling. For the most part, using the *most current* drug reference book will keep you up to date.

You will recognize the schedule of a particular controlled substance by noting a *C* with either *I, II, III, IV,* or *V* after it. Some references show the capital *C* with the Roman numeral inside the curve of the *C* (Ⓒ). Labels on controlled substances are also designated with a *C* and a Roman numeral to indicate its level of control. Drug inserts (information leaflets accompanying drugs) are also marked with a *C* and the appropriate schedule number. (See Figure 1.1 and Table 1.1.)

TABLE 1.1. FIVE SCHEDULES OF CONTROLLED SUBSTANCES

Schedule Number	Abuse Potential and Legal Limitations	Examples of Substances
1, Ⓒ	High abuse potential Limited medical use	heroin, LSD, marijuana, mescaline
2, Ⓒ	High abuse potential May lead to severe dependence Written prescription only No phoning in of prescription by office health worker No refills In emergency, physician may phone in, but handwritten prescription must go to pharmacy within 72 hours	morphine, codeine, Demerol, methadone, Percodan, Dilaudid, Ritalin, cocaine
3, Ⓒ	May lead to limited dependence Written or verbal (phoned in) prescription, by physician only May be refilled up to five times in 6 months	paregoric, Noludar, Empirin with codeine, aspirin with codeine, Fiorinal
4, Ⓒ	Lower abuse potential than the above schedules Prescription may be written out by health care worker, but must be signed by physician Prescription may be phoned in by health care worker May be refilled up to five times in 6 months	Valium, Placidyl, chloral hydrate, phenobarbital, Librium, Darvon, Dalmane
5, Ⓒ	Low abuse potential compared to the above schedules Depending on *state* law, may require a prescription or may be sold over the counter; purchaser must be 18 years old and sign a form (Exempt Narcotic Registration Form) with the pharmacist Consists primarily of preparations for cough suppressants containing codeine and preparations for diarrhea (e.g., paregoric, an opium tincture)	Cheracol syrup, Robitussin-DAC, Dimetane Expectorant DC, Donnagel-PG, Lomotil

8

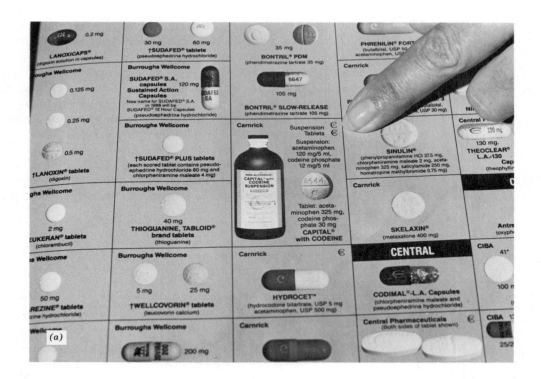

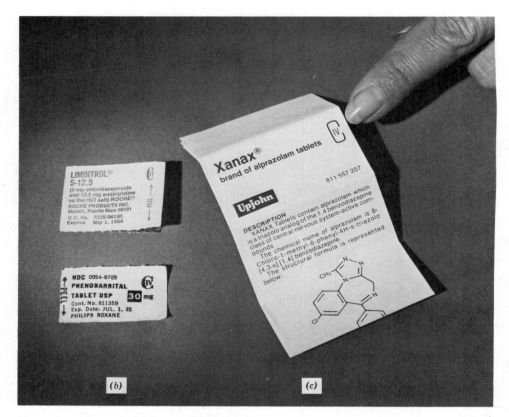

Figure 1.1 *Controlled substance schedule numbers appear in a variety of drug information resources, including (a) the Physician's Desk Reference, (b) drug packages, and (c) drug inserts.*

FDA and DEA

The increase in the number of drugs produced for marketing brought dangers to the public. The federal Food and Drug Administration was established to assure that some basic standards would be followed. Its responsibilities include:

- Inspecting plants where foods, drugs, or cosmetics are made
- Reviewing new drug applications and petitions for food additives
- Investigating and removing unsafe drugs from the market
- Assuring proper labeling of foods, cosmetics, and drugs

When the need for better control of addictive drugs became urgent, the FDA had its hands full just trying to enforce basic drug standards. It became imperative to set up a new department, the Drug Enforcement Administration, in 1970 to handle all the needs and safety controls for the more dangerous drugs. Thus, the two agencies — FDA and DEA — were established with their own specific areas of drug control.

As a health care worker and an informed citizen, you must keep informed of the latest developments concerning these two agencies. Hardly a week goes by without mention of the activities of the FDA or the DEA in the news. You should be able to recognize their separate areas of control.

FDA

Concerned with general safety standards in the production of drugs, foods, and cosmetics

Responsible for approval and removal of products on the market

DEA

Concerned with controlled substances only

Enforces laws against drug activities, including illegal drug use, dealing, and manufacturing

Monitors need for changing the schedules of abused drugs

Health Care Workers and the Law

In some ways, you will be as involved as the physician in observing the restrictions of the drug laws. You will have the responsibility of keeping accurate records of the medications dispensed. You will maintain the supply of drugs at your facility. If you work in a doctor's office, you also will be involved with phoning in prescriptions and securing prescription forms at your facility.

The following guidelines should be followed by the health care worker involved in dispensing medications:

1. Keep a current drug reference book available at all times. You should be able to readily identify substances that must be controlled.

2. Keep controlled substances locked securely. Double-locking is recommended. This means:
   a. Placing the drugs in a locked safety box
   b. Placing the locked box in a cupboard that is also locked

3. Conceal prescription pads at your office, clinic, or facility. Do not leave pads out in the open, especially in patient examining rooms. The prescription pads, with the physician's DEA registration number, are a possible source of fraud and drug tampering when forged and used illegally. Keep the pads in a designated location (e.g., a drawer), out of the public areas of the office or nursing station.

4. Keep accurate records of each controlled substance dispensed, received, or destroyed at your facility. These records, as well as the records from the previous 2 years, must be available at all times.

5. Be responsible for keeping up to date with current news of the activities of the FDA and the DEA. Keep informed of any changes in the scheduling of controlled substances.

6. Establish a working rapport with a pharmacist. A local pharmacist is an excellent resource for you when you are unsure of your legal responsibilities with drugs or have any uncertainties about drug therapy.

7. If you work in an office, maintain a professional rapport with the pharmaceutical representatives who leave drug samples there. They are also excellent resources of drug information.

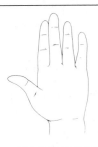

STOP!
Check your knowledge of this chapter before going any further.

CHAPTER REVIEW QUIZ

Complete the following statements:

1. The first major U.S. drug law was passed in the year _____ and was called the _____ .

2. *USP* stands for _____ and is the title of _____ .

3. *NF* stands for _____ .

4. Which drug law established the *USP* and *NF* (which are now one)?
   _____

5. The agency that requires you to keep a record of each controlled substance transaction is the _____ .

6. Prescriptions for schedule C-_____ drugs may be phoned in by the health care worker.

7. In some states, an Exempt Narcotic Registration Form need only be signed at the pharmacy to obtain drugs in the C-_____ schedule.

8. How long must you keep an inventory record of each controlled substance transaction at your office? _____

9. Three responsibilities of the FDA include:

   _____

   _____

   _____

10. What types of drugs are listed in the C-V schedule?
    _____

11. What method is recommended for securing the controlled substances at your office? _____

12. If a patient calls to request a refill of a Percodan (C-II) prescription, how would you reply?
    _____

2

Drug Names and References

OBJECTIVES

Upon completion of this chapter, the student will be able to:

1. Define the following as they relate to drugs: pharmacology, classification, prototype, action, indication, adverse reaction, precautions, interactions, and contraindications.
2. Differentiate among the following drug names: generic name, official name, trade name, and chemical name.
3. Explain what is indicated by a number included in a drug trade name (e.g., Phenaphen No. 3).
4. Define and explain the restrictions of drug sales implied by the following: OTC, legend drug, and controlled substance.
5. List at least two drug references available today.
6. Discuss several characteristics that *you* consider important in choosing the best drug reference.
7. Identify the types of information listed on drug cards.
8. Define the following side effects: ototoxicity, nephrotoxicity, tinnitus, and photosensitivity.

Pharmacology can be defined as the study of drugs and their origin, nature, properties, and effects upon living organisms. We need to know why drugs are given, how they work, and what effects to expect. The thousands of drugs products on the market would make this subject difficult to tackle if it were not for:

- Numerous drug references, geared to a variety of levels of readers, from laypersons to pharmacists
- Grouping of drugs under broad subcategories
- Continuity in the use of basic identifying terms for the names and actions of drugs

Classifications

Each drug can be categorized under a broad subcategory, or subcategories, called *classifications* (see list below). Drugs that affect the body in similar ways are listed in the same classification. Drugs that have several types of therapeutic effects fit under several classifications. For example, aspirin has a variety of effects on the body. It may be given to relieve pain (analgesic), to reduce fever (antipyretic), or to reduce inflammation of tissues (anti-inflammatory). Therefore, aspirin is categorized under three classifications of drugs (as shown in parentheses).

Another drug, cyclobenzaprine (Flexeril), however, is known to be used for only one therapeutic effect: to relieve muscle spasms. Flexeril, therefore, is listed under only one classification (muscle relaxant).

Examples of some of the other drug classifications are listed below. Are you familiar with any of them already?

adrenergics	cholinergics	hormones
anesthetics	decongestants	hypnotics
antibiotics	diuretics	laxatives
antihistamines	electrolytes	sedatives
antihypertensives	emetics	tranquilizers
antitussives	expectorants	vasoconstrictors
cardiotonics	hematinics	vasodilators

The second part of this text compares the characteristics of the various major drug classifications. In each chapter, as a classification is explained, you will learn what general information to associate with drugs of that classification:

- Therapeutic uses
- Most common side effects
- Precautions to be used
- Contraindications
- Interactions that may occur when taken with other drugs or foods
- Some of the most common product names, usual dosages, and comments on administration

You will also be given a prototype of each classification. A *prototype* is a model example, a drug that typifies the characteristics of that classification. Hopefully, each time you learn of a new drug, you will associate the prototype and its characteristics with the new drug, based on its classification.

You can find the classification, as well as the various names of the drug, by referring to a drug reference book.

Identifying Names

Four terms apply to the various titles of a drug:

1. *Generic name.* Common or general name assigned to the drug; differentiated from trade name by initial lowercase letter; never capitalized
2. *Trade name.* The name by which a pharmaceutical company identifies its product; is copyrighted and used exclusively by that company; can be distinguished from generic name by capitalized first letter and is often shown on labels and references with the symbol ® behind the name (for "registered" trademark)
3. *Chemical name.* The exact molecular formula of the drug; usually a long, very difficult name to pronounce and of no concern to the health care worker
4. *Official name.* Name of the drug as it appears in the official reference, the *USP/NF*; generally the same as the generic name

The use of generic and trade names for drugs can be compared to the various names of grocery products. Two examples of generic names are orange juice and detergent. Corresponding trade names are Sunkist, Bird's Eye, Tropicana, and Minute Maid, and Cheer, Tide, All, and Fab. While there is only one generic name, there may be many trade names.

When a company produces a new drug for the market, it assigns a generic name to the product. After testing and approval by the FDA, the drug company gives the drug a trade name (often something short and easy to remember when advertised). For 17 years, the company has the exclusive right to market the drug. Once approved, the drug is listed in the *USP/NF* by an official name, which is usually the same as the generic name. When 17 years have passed, other companies may begin to combine the same chemicals to form that specific generic product for marketing. Each company will assign their own specific trade name to the product.

Compare the names of the following two drugs:

Generic Name	Chemical Name	Trade Name (Drug Company)
tetracycline hydrochloride	4-dimethylamino-4,12 aocta-hydro-3,6,10,12,12a pentahydroxyl-6-methyl-1,11-dioxi-2 naphthacenecarboxamide hydrochloride	Achromycin (Lederle Labs) Sumycin (Squibb) Tetracyn (Pfipharmecs) Tetracycline HCL (Premo Labs)*

*Some companies simply elect to market the product by the generic name.

Generic Name	Chemical Name	Trade Name (Drug Company)
propoxyphene hydrochloride	alpha-4-dimethylamino-3-methyl-1,2-diphenyl-2 butanol, proprionate hydrochloride	Darvon (Eli Lilly) Propoxyphene HCL (Rexall)*

PATIENT EDUCATION

Patients may ask you about the difference between generic and trade (brand) name products. Generally, trade name products are more expensive, although the basic active ingredients (drug contents) are the same as in the generic. The higher price helps to pay for advertisements promoting the trade name. (Can you think of certain trade names that are heavily advertised in television commercials?)

For this reason it is economically wise to compare prices of over-the-counter (OTC) products that have the same generic components and strengths. For example, several cough syrups may have exactly the same contents, but the prices may vary widely.

Concerning prescription drugs, most states have enacted legislation encouraging physicians to let pharmacists substitute less expensive *generic equivalents* for prescribed brand name drugs. Specific provisions of *drug substitution laws* vary from state to state.

The physician may indicate "no substitutions" on the prescription. Often physicians have preferences for certain products. Even though the drug contents are the same, the "fillers," or ingredients that are used to hold the preparation together, may be slightly different. This difference in fillers may affect how quickly the drug dissolves or takes effect. Dyes in some products may alter effects in some sensitive patients by leading to an allergic response.

Many products are combinations of several generic components. You will recognize this when you see several generic names (not capitalized) and corresponding amounts listed under one trade name (capitalized). Examples are:

Trade Name	Generic Name and Amount
Darvocet-N-100	acetaminophen, 650 mg propoxyphene napsylate, 100 mg
Darvon Compound-65	aspirin, 227 mg propoxyphene HCL, 65 mg caffeine, 32 mg
Ornade	chlorpheniramine, 8 mg isopropanolamine iodide, 2.5 mg phenylpropanolamine, 50 mg

It should be noted that a number may be part of the trade name. The number often refers to an amount of one of the generic components and helps to differentiate it from an almost identical product. Identify the significance of the numbers in comparing the following trade names:

Trade Name	Generic Name and Amount
Empirin	aspirin, 325 mg
Empirin No. 1	aspirin, 325 mg codeine phosphate, 7.5 mg

*Some companies simply elect to market the product by the generic name.

Trade Name	Generic Name and Amount
Empirin No. 2	aspirin, 325 mg
	codeine phosphate, 15 mg
Empirin No. 3	aspirin, 325 mg
	codeine phosphate, 30 mg
Empirin No. 4	aspirin, 325 mg
	codeine phosphate, 60 mg

While one of the products is plain aspirin, the other four have a controlled substance, codeine, added. *The larger the number, the greater the amount of controlled substance present.* Other trade names including numbers which can also be written in this way, include:

Fiorinal #1, #2, #3
Tylenol #1, #2, #3, #4
Phenaphen #2, #3, #4

Many drug errors have occurred because the trade name was misinterpreted for the number of tablets to be given. So . . .

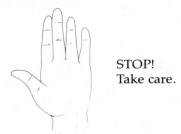

STOP!
Take care.

Be certain you can clearly read and understand the order!

Another type of drug error involves needless allergic reactions to one of the generic components of a medication. The problem stems from:

Not consulting the patient's chart for the history of allergies before a new medication is ordered or given

Not checking a reference to find out if a medication being ordered or given contains any generic components to which the patient has a known allergy

For example, if a patient has an allergy to aspirin, do not administer the first dose of any new medication to the patient without finding out if the product contains aspirin. Although the doctor is in error for ordering the medication, you are also in error for administering a medication with which you are unfamiliar. The physician is often hurried and pressured in meeting the demands of an office schedule. A proficient health care worker should check the history and chart for known allergies, and pick up any discrepancies. Alertness is the key to an efficient clinic, institution, or facility.

Always keep a drug reference handy, and use it when you are unfamiliar with the generic components of a drug ordered for a patient with known drug allergies. With experience, you will learn and remember the names of products most commonly used at your facility.

Legal Terms Referring to Drugs

A drug may be referred to by terms other than its classification, generic name, trade name, chemical name, or official name. As mentioned in Chapter 1, the following terms imply the legal accessibility of the drug:

1. *OTC.* Over-the-counter; no purchasing restrictions by the FDA
2. *Legend drug.* Prescription drug; determined unsafe for over-the-counter purchase because of possible harmful side effects if taken indiscriminantly; includes birth control pills, antibiotics, cardiac drugs, hormones, etc.; indicated in the *Physician's Desk Reference* (discussed later in this chapter) by the symbol ℞ to the far right of the trade name
3. *Controlled substance.* Drug controlled by prescription requirement because of the danger of addiction or abuse; indicated in references by schedule numbers C-I to C-V (see Chapter 1)

Terms Indicating Drug Actions

Most references follow a similar format in describing drugs. When you research drug information, you will find the following terms as headings under each drug. You will find specific information more quickly if you understand what is listed under each heading.

Indications. A list of medical conditions or diseases for which the drug is meant to be used (e.g., Benadryl, a trade name, diphenhydramine hydrochloride, is a commonly used drug; indications include allergic rhinitis, mild allergic skin reactions, motion sickness, and mild cases of parkinsonism).

Actions. A description of the cellular changes that occur as a result of the drug. This information tends to be very technical, describing cellular and tissue changes. While it is helpful to know what body system is affected by the drug, this information is geared more for the pharmacist (e.g., as an antihistamine, Benadryl appears to compete with histamine for cell receptor sites on effector cells).

Contraindications. A list of conditions for which the drug should *not* be given (e.g., two common contraindications for Benadryl are pregnancy or lactating mother).

Warnings and Precautions. A list of conditions or types of patients that warrant closer observation for specific side effects when given the drug (e.g., due to atropinelike activity, Benadryl must be used cautiously with patients who have a history of bronchial asthma, hypertension, or increased intraocular pressure).

Side Effects and Adverse Reactions. A list of possible unpleasant or dangerous secondary effects, other than the desired effect (e.g., side effects of Benadryl include sedation, dizziness, disturbed coordination, epigastric distress, anorexia, and thickening of bronchial secretions). This listing may be

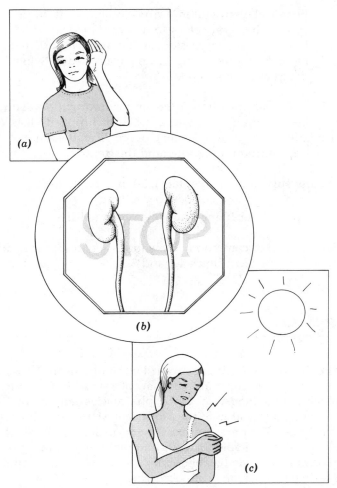

Figure 2.1 *Side effects or adverse reactions can include* (a) *ototoxicity,* (b) *nephrotoxicity, and* (c) *photosensitivity.*

quite extensive, with as many as 50 or more side effects for one drug. Because it is difficult to know which are *most* likely to occur, choose a reference book that underlines or italicizes the most common side effects. Certain drugs may have side effects with which you are not familiar. Note the definitions of the following three side effects associated with specific antibiotics (see Fig. 2.1):

- Ototoxicity causes damage to the eighth cranial nerve, resulting in impaired hearing or ringing in the ears (tinnitus). Damage may be reversible or permanent.
- Nephrotoxicity causes damage to the kidneys, resulting in impaired kidney function, decreased output, and renal failure.
- Photosensitivity is an increased reaction to sunlight, with the danger of intense sunburn.

Interactions. A list of other drugs or foods which may alter the effect of the drug, and usually should *not* be given during the same course of therapy (e.g., monoamine oxidase (MAO) inhibitors will intensify the effects of

Benadryl; you will find MAO inhibitors listed under interactions for many drugs; the term refers to a group of drugs that have been used for the treatment of depression; it has been found that they can cause serious blood pressure changes, and even death, when taken with many other drugs and some foods).

Other headings often listed under information about a drug include "How Supplied" and "Usual Dosage." "How Supplied" lists the available forms and strengths of the drug. "Usual Dosage" lists the amount of drug considered safe for administration, the route, and the frequency of administration. For example:

How supplied: tablets (tabs): 20 mg and 40 mg
suppository, 20 mg
Usual dosage: 10 mg orally every 4 h (q4h)

For a listing of common abbreviations regarding drug administration and medication orders, see Tables 4.1 and 5.1.

Drug References*

The *Physician's Desk Reference (PDR)* is one of the most widely used references for drugs in current use. It is an old standby found in every medical setting: offices, clinics, hospital units, pharmacies, and so on. As the name indicates, however, it is geared to the physician. Many new choices of references are available today. Four are compared here, including the *PDR*. You must find the reference most suitable for you, one that you can interpret quickly and easily. By becoming knowledgeable about the drugs you administer, you may prevent possible drug errors from occurring.

Physician's Desk Reference (PDR)†

Pro	Con
Distributed to practicing physicians; single hardback volume	Geared for physicians and pharmacists
Several supplements published throughout the year, with revised information or descriptions of new products introduced after the previous edition went to press	Lengthy descriptions
	Difficult to sort out what is most important to remember
	No easily identified nursing implications
All drugs cross-referenced, by several color-coded indexes, according to one of the following:	Includes many code numbers in the description of "How Supplied," making it difficult to interpret
• Company that makes the drug (white, "Manufacturers' Index")	Contains only those drugs that manufacturers pay to have
• Trade name (pink, "Product Name Index")	incorporated; incomplete with regard to OTC drugs, making it

*References listed here were used to compile the information in this book.
†Published annually by Biomedical Information Corp., New York, New York.

Pro	*Con*

Pro

- Drug classification (blue, Product Classification Index)
- Generic name (yellow, "Generic and Chemical Name Index")

Includes photographs of many drugs

Includes a list of all U.S. Poison Control Centers, with addresses and phone numbers

Includes a description of substances used for medical testing (green, "Diagnostic Product Information"), for example, barium, X-ray dyes, substances used for allergy testing

Con

necessary to buy *PDR* OTC book

*United States Pharmacopeia/Dispensing Information (USP/DI)**

Pro

Two paperback volumes (and six updates on new drugs per year):
- *Drug Information for the Health Provider,* drug information for the physician; includes up-to-date information on carcinogenicity (studies on the ability of drugs to cause cancer)
- *Advice for the Patient*

Easy-to-read, practical guidelines for the patient

Stresses most important aspects of the patient's history for the physician to be aware of before prescribing the drug

Stresses many tips for proper use of medication and what precautions to take

Includes a pronunciation key for each drug name

Con

No photographs of drugs

Must be purchased, is not distributed freely

American Hospital Formulary Service†

Pro

Distributed to practicing physicians; single paperback volume

Good, concise information; easy to read

Con

Some parts (e.g., "Chemical Information" and "Drug Stability") not necessary for the health care worker

---

*Published annually by U.S. Pharmacopeial Convention, Inc., Rockville, Maryland.
†Published by the American Society of Hospital Pharmacists, Bethesda, Maryland.

Pro	Con
Arranged by classifications, with a general statement about each classification at the beginning of each section	Does not clearly identify controlled substance schedule numbers

Compendium of Drug Therapy*

Pro	Con
Distributed to practicing physicians; two hardback volumes: • *Compendium of Patient Information,* helpful patient guidelines for a particular specialty area (e.g., obstetrics, orthopedics, pediatrics, family practice, etc.) • *Compendium of Drug Therapy* Very easy to read, well arranged Index tabs easily separate sections by drug classification Includes photographs of drugs Includes phone numbers of major pharmaceutical companies and Poison Control Centers Includes copies of some drug package inserts	None

Other references (e.g., *The Pill Book, Handbook of Nonprescription Drugs*) may be found in bookstores, but they may not contain adequate information for the health care worker. Your school may recommend a specific drug reference other than the four listed in this text. Many new references geared to the nurse or health care worker are currently being published.

Drug Cards

As a student of pharmacology, you may find it helpful to prepare drug cards because there are so many drugs to learn. Many educational programs require drug cards with the curriculum. You may use 3 × 5 or 5 × 7 -inch index cards stored in a recipe card box or other similar file. Included on the cards should be the information most useful to medical personnel. Although the cards should be updated periodically, using them saves valuable time compared to using the larger drug references. Certain information should be included on the drug card:

1. Generic and trade name of the drug
2. Classification or classifications of the drug
3. Forms in which the drug is available

*Published annually by Biomedical Information Corp., New York, New York.

4. Drug action
5. Indications
6. Side effects
7. Routes of administration
8. Dosage range and customary dosage
9. Any special instructions for giving the medication

In addition to making it easier and faster to locate information on drugs, drug cards constitute an ideal method of becoming more knowledgeable about drugs, classifications, and other pharmaceutical terminology.

Pharmaceutical salespeople and drug company representatives frequently have drug inserts or package brochures that are also useful. Such material can be attached to index cards or filed separately. It is especially important that drug cards be prepared on those drugs used predominantly at your medical facility.

The following is a sample drug card. Note that a number of abbreviations are used to save space. Common abbreviations regarding drug administration and medication orders appear in Tables 4.1 and 5.1.

Drug. Nitroglycerin (Nitro-Bid, Nitrostat)

Classification. Vasodilator.

Form. Sublingual tablet, timed-release tablets or capsules, ointment, dermal patches, and IV.

Action. Relaxes smooth muscles, dilates arterioles and capillaries.

Uses. Management of acute angina pectoris episodes.

Side Effects and Toxicities. Headache with throbbing, dizziness, weakness, blurred vision, dry mouth, and tachycardia.

Route. Sublingual, topical, by mouth (PO), or IV.

Dosage. Sublingual, one tablet under tongue or in buccal pouch, may be repeated three times (×3) if necessary; timed-release capsule, two or three times a day at 8–12-h intervals; ointment, apply to any convenient skin area and spread in thin, uniform layer 1–2 inches, may be applied every 3–4 h (q3–4h) whenever necessary (PRN).

Special Instruction. Severe headache may occur; flushing, dizziness, or weakness is usually transient; if blurred vision or dry mouth occurs, discontinue use.

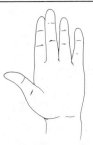

STOP!
Check your knowledge of this chapter before going any further.

CHAPTER REVIEW QUIZ

Match the definition with the term:

1. _____ List of conditions for which a drug is meant to be used

2. _____ Subcategories of drugs, based on their effects on the body

3. _____ Description of the cellular changes that occur as a result of a drug

4. _____ Conditions for which a drug should not be given

a. Contraindications
b. Precautions
c. Indications
d. Prototype
e. Actions
f. Classifications

Refer to the following drug description to answer questions 5–8:

Pyridium®   ℞
(phenazopyridine HCl tablets, USP)
Product of Warner-Lambert, Inc.
Description: Pyridium (phenozopyridine HCl) is a urinary tract analgesic agent, chemically designated 2.6-pyridinediamine, 3-(phenylazo), monohydrochloride.

5. The generic name of the drug is _____ .

6. The chemical name of the drug is _____ .

7. The trade name of the drug is _____ .

8. What is indicated by the ℞ symbol in the upper right corner?
   _____ .

9. List four drug references:

   _____   _____

   _____   _____

10. Explain the difference between these two medication orders:

    a. Give two Empirin, PO.

    b. Give one Empirin #2, PO.

    _____

    _____

3

Sources and Bodily Effects of Drugs

OBJECTIVES

Upon completion of this chapter, the student will be able to:

1. Identify the four sources of drugs.
2. Differentiate between the following: drug actions and drug effects, systemic effects and local effects, loading dose and maintenance dose, and toxic dose and lethal dose.
3. Define the following processes as they are related to the passage of drugs through the body. Give conditions that may decrease the effectiveness of each: absorption, distribution, metabolism, and excretion.
4. Define the following terms: selective distribution, toxicity, placebo, synergism, potentiation, and antagonism.
5. List several variables that may affect the action of drugs.
6. Identify the fastest route of drug administration.
7. Define the following undesirable drug effects: teratogenic effect, idiosyncracy, tolerance, dependence, hypersensitivity, and anaphylactic reaction.

Sources of Drugs

Any chemical substance taken into the body for the purpose of affecting body function is referred to as a *drug*. In earlier times, these substances were found in nature, sometimes accidentally. *Plants* were the primary source of substances used on the human body. Berries, bark, leaves, resin from trees, and roots were found to aid the body and are still very important drug sources today.

Minerals from the earth and soil also found their way into human use as drugs. Iron, sulfur, potassium, silver, and even gold are some of the minerals used to prepare drugs.

More sophisticated sources of drugs emerged as human beings progressed. Research led to the use of substances from *animals* as effective drugs. Substances lacking in the human body can be replaced with similar substances from the glands, organs, and tissues of animals. The origin of drugs from an animal source even now includes human extractions. The pituitary gland from cadavers can be used to make a drug for the treatment of growth disorders.

Finally, chemists use *synthetic* sources to make drugs to market for human consumption. The synthetic (manufactured) sources evolved with human skills in laboratories and advanced understanding of chemistry. Drug compounds are produced from artificial rather than natural substances. This method is probably the most actively pursued source of drugs by major companies today. Competitive research is a big industry in experimenting with chemicals to discover cures for current medical problems. Numerous antibiotics are synthetic or semisynthetic, the results of researchers' meeting the need for better treatment of infections. Someday the cure for cancer may be found from a synthetic source developed in a laboratory.

Two exciting developments in drug research occurred during the 1980s:

- The Eli Lilly company developed a new insulin that does not require an animal source. Humulin, which is more similar to human insulin than its predecessors, is made from *Escherichia coli* bacteria and altered DNA molecules.
- The Discovery III space shuttle, launched in August 1984, carried the first nonastronaut space traveler. On board, a researcher conducted experiments with a drug processing machine. The ongoing goal of the space research is to produce a degree of drug purity that cannot be attained under conditions influenced by gravity.

Effects of Drugs

No matter how different the sources, the common characteristic of all drugs is the ability to affect body function in some manner. When introduced into the body, all drugs cause cellular changes (drug actions), followed by some physiological change (drug effect). Generally, drug effects may be categorized as systemic or local:

SOURCES OF DRUGS:

	EXAMPLE:	TRADE NAME:	CLASSIFICATION:
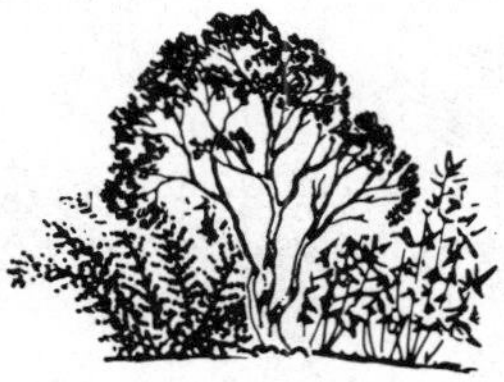 **PLANTS**	cinchona bark	Quinidine	antiarrhthymic
	purple foxglove plant	Digitalis	cardiotonic
	poppy plant (opium)	Paregoric, Morphine Codeine	antidiarrheal analgesic analgesic, antitussive
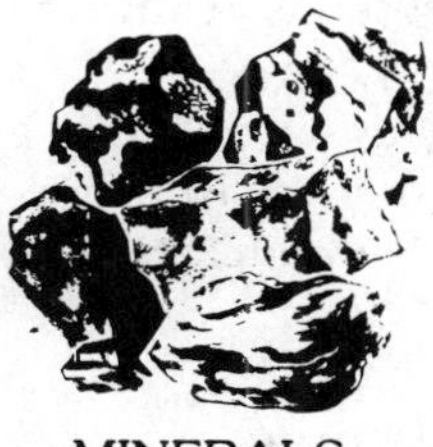 **MINERALS**	magnesium	Milk of Magnesia	antacid, laxative
	silver	Silver Nitrate	ophthalmic anti-infective (eye drops placed in the eyes of newborns)
	gold	Solganal, Auranofin	anti-inflammatory; used in the treatment of rheumatoid arthritis
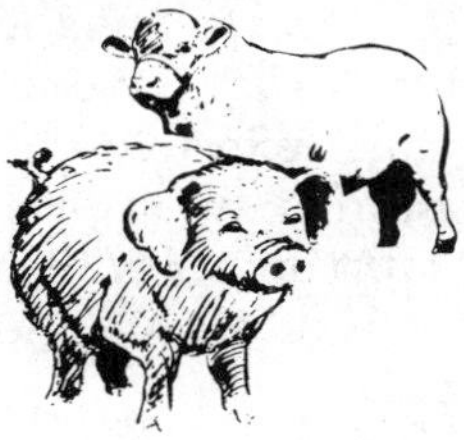 **ANIMALS**	pancreas of cow, hog	Insulin	antidiabetic hormone
	stomach of cow, hog	Pepsin	digestive hormone
	thyroid gland of animals	Thyroid, USP	hormone
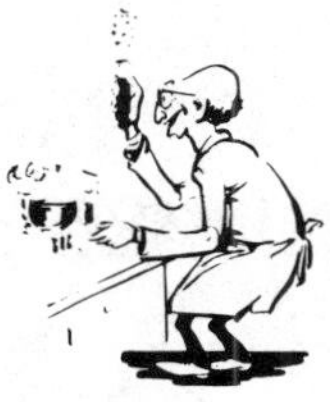 **SYNTHETIC**	meperidine	Demerol	analgesic
	diphenoxylate	Lomotil	antidiarrheal
	sulfisoxazole	Gantrisin	anti-infective sulfonamide; used in the treatment of urinary tract infections

Figure 3.1 *Sources of drugs.* (a) *Plant sources;* (b) *mineral sources;* (c) *animal sources;* (d) *synthetic sources.*

1. *Systemic effect.* Reaches widespread areas of the body (e.g., acetaminophen (Tylenol) suppository, although given rectally, has the ability to be absorbed and distributed throughout the body to cause a general reduction in fever and pain).
2. *Local effect.* Is limited to the area of the body where it is administered (e.g., dibucaine oint (Nupercainal), applied rectally, affects only the rectal mucosa to reduce hemorrhoidal pain).

Drug Processing by the Body

Within the body, drugs undergo several changes. From start to finish, the biological changes consist of four processes:

1. *Absorption.* Getting into the bloodstream.
2. *Distribution.* Moving from the bloodstream into the tissues and fluids of the body.
3. *Metabolism.* Physical and chemical alterations that a substance undergoes in the body.
4. *Excretion.* Eliminating waste products of drug metabolism from the body.

Many variables affect how quickly or successfully substances go through the body via these four processes. If any of the four processes is hampered, the drug action and affects will be hampered. Note in Table 3.1 conditions that may hamper each process.

Directions for the administration of one drug versus another may vary widely because the physical properties of the drugs may vary widely. The specific directions ("Usual Dosage and Administration," "Contraindications," and "Warnings") that accompany each drug are given to enhance the absorption, distribution, metabolism, and excretion of the drug. For example, directions to "Give on an empty stomach" ensure the most effective means of absorption. "Use cautiously in patients with renal dysfunction" implies possible effects on the excretion of a drug. "Decrease dose in patients with hepatic dysfunction" implies possible effects on the metabolism of a drug. *Read all labels carefully, and caution the patient to do so also* (See Fig. 3.2).

TABLE 3.1. PROCESSING OF DRUGS WITHIN THE BODY

Process	Primary Site of Process	Conditions That May Hamper Process
Absorption	Mucosa of the stomach, mouth, small intestine, or rectum; blood vessels in the muscles or subcutaneous tissues; or dermal layers	Incorrect administration may destroy the drug before it reaches the bloodstream or its site of action (e.g., giving antibiotics after meals instead of on an empty stomach).
Distribution	Circulatory system, through capillaries and across cell membranes	Poor circulation (impaired flow of blood) may prevent drug from reaching tissues.
Metabolism	Liver	Hepatitis, cirrhosis of liver, or a damaged liver may prevent adequate breakdown of drug, thus causing a buildup of unmetabolized drug.
Excretion	Kidneys, sweat glands, lungs, breast milk, feces, or bile	Renal damage or kidney failure may prevent passage of drug waste products, thereby causing an accumulation of the drug in the body.

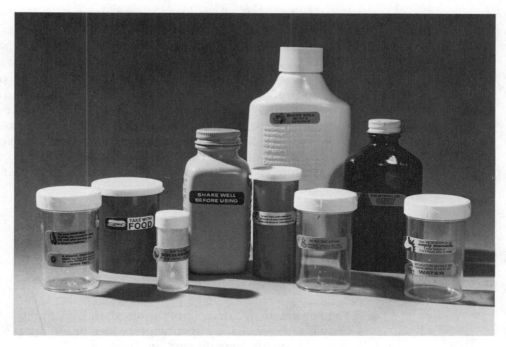

Figure 3.2   *Read labels carefully before administration.*

Absorption

The site of absorption of drugs varies according to the following physical properties of each drug:

1. *pH.* Drugs of a slightly acidic nature (e.g., aspirin and tetracycline) are absorbed well through the stomach mucosa. Drugs of an alkaline pH are not absorbed well through the stomach, but are readily absorbed in the alkaline environment of the small intestine. The antibiotic tetracycline is recommended to be given on an empty stomach so that its pH is not altered. If given an the presence of milk, dairy products, or antacids, it will not be properly absorbed. Oral medications for infants (syrups and solutions) may not be absorbed well after infant feedings. The milk or formula neutralizes the acidity of the stomach. Thus, absorption may be enhanced when the infant is given medications on an empty stomach.

2. *Lipid (fat) solubility.* Substances high in lipid solubility are quickly and easily absorbed through the mucosa of the stomach. Alcohol and substances containing alcohol are soluble in lipids. They are rapidly absorbed through the gastrointestinal (GI) tract. Substances low in lipid solubility are not absorbed well through the stomach or intestinal mucosa, and are absorbed best when given by a means other than the GI tract. An exception is the drug neomycin, which is not lipid soluble and yet is given orally. It is indicated for suppression of intestinal bacteria before intestinal or bowel

surgery, or in the treatment of bacterial diarrhea. By giving neomycin orally, it passes through the GI tract, unable to be absorbed. As a result, it tends to build up and accumulate in the bowel. There, the trapped antibiotic kills the bacteria in the bowel, for the desired effect.

3. *Presence or absence of food in the stomach.* Food in the stomach tends to slow absorption due to a slower emptying of the stomach. If a fast drug effect is desired, an empty stomach will facilitate quicker absorption. On the other hand, giving some medications on an empty stomach is contraindicated. Medications that are irritating to the stomach can be buffered by the presence of food. Directions may indicate "Give before meals" or "Take with food" to decrease side effects (e.g., nausea and gastric ulcers) on the GI tract.

Distribution

The movement of a drug from the bloodstream into the tissues and fluids of the body is also affected by specific properties of the drug. Reaching sites beyond the major organs may depend on the drug's ability to cross a lipid membrane. Some drugs pass the "blood-brain barrier" or the "placental barrier," while others do not. You may read about drugs contraindicated for lactating mothers because the drug has the ability to pass through the cell membranes into the milk.

Some drugs have a *selective distribution* (see Fig. 3.3). This refers to an affinity, or attraction, of a drug to a specific organ or cells. For example, amphetamines have a selective distribution to cerebrospinal fluid (CSF). The human chorionic gonadotropin (HCG) hormone, which is used as a fertility drug, has a selective distribution to the ovaries.

By virtue of their properties, some drugs are distributed more slowly than others. Thus, while two drugs may be categorized in the same drug classification, one may be known to act on the cells and achieve the effect more quickly than the other.

Metabolism

When transformed in the liver, a drug is broken down and altered to more water-soluble by-products. Thus, the drug may be more easily excreted by the kidneys.

If hepatic disease is present, a patient may exhibit toxic (poisonous) effects of a drug. This occurs because the drug is not being broken down properly by the inefficient liver. It may accumulate, unchanged by the liver, and may be unable to pass out of the body's excretory system.

It is possible for some drugs to bypass the process of metabolism. They reach the kidney virtually unchanged and may later be detected in the urine.

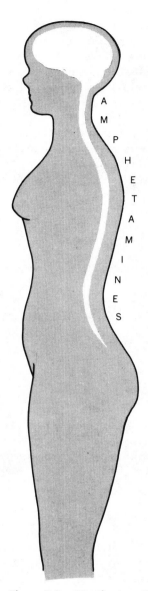

Figure 3.3   *Distribution. One example of selective distribution is the attraction of amphetamines to the cerebrospinal fluid.*

Excretion

While it is possible for some drugs to be eliminated through the lungs (e.g., exhaled gases and anesthetics) or through perspiration, feces, bile, or breast milk, most are excreted by the kidneys.

If a drug is not excreted properly before repeated doses are given, eventually a cumulative effect may occur. A *cumulative effect* is an increased effect of a drug demonstrated when repeated doses accumulate in the body. If unnoticed, the cumulative effect may build to a dangerous, or toxic, level.

Toxicity refers to a condition that results from exposure to either a poison or a dangerous amount of a drug, that is normally safe when given in a smaller amount. In drug therapy, the goal is to give just enough of the drug to cause the desired (therapeutic) effect while keeping the amount below the level at which toxic effects are observed.

Digoxin is a cardiac drug which must be given cautiously because of its potential for causing a cumulative effect. Normally, digoxin slows the heart rate, but if the drug accumulates, the heart rate may slow to a dangerously low level. Circulation and renal function must be adequate, or the digoxin will accumulate, leading to digoxin toxicity.

Other Variables

Many variables affect the speed and efficiency of drugs being processed by the body. The physical properties of the drugs themselves and the condition of the body systems have been discussed. Other variables affecting drug action and effect follow.

AGE

Metabolism and excretion are slower in the elderly, and therefore attention must be paid to possible cumulative effects. Children have a lower threshold of response and react more rapidly and sometimes in unexpected ways; therefore, frequent assessment is imperative.

WEIGHT

Generally, the bigger the person, the greater the dose should be. However, there is great individual variation in sensitivity to drugs. Many drug dosages are always calculated on the basis of the patient's weight.

SEX

Women respond differently than men to some drugs. The ratio of fat per body mass differs, and so do hormone levels. If the female is pregnant or nursing, most drugs are contraindicated, or the dosage must be adjusted.

PSYCHOLOGICAL STATE

It has been proven that the more positive the patient feels about the medication he or she is taking, the more positive the physical response. This is referred to as the *placebo effect*.

A *placebo* is an inactive substance that resembles a medication, although no drug is present. For example, a sugar tablet or a saline solution for injection may be used as a placebo.

Placebos are most often used in "blind study" experiments, in which groups of people are given either a drug or a placebo. The individuals, unaware of which they have been given, are studied for the effects. Often, by virtue of strong belief, the placebo-administered individuals achieve the desired effect associated with the drug they think they have received.

Placebos are occasionally given to patients who are developing a psychological dependence on a drug. Substituting a placebo for the drug may prevent a physical dependence.

It is also possible to have a decreased drug effect when the attitude of a patient toward a medication is negative.

 The significance for you, the health care worker, is to recognize that your attitude regarding a medication may be picked up by the patient and indirectly affect the patient's response to the drug.

DRUG INTERACTIONS

Whenever more than one drug is taken, it is possible that the combination may alter the normal expected response of each individual drug. One drug may interact with another to increase, decrease, or cancel out the effects of the other.

The following terms are used to describe drug interactions:

Synergism. The action of two drugs working together in which one helps the other simultaneously for an effect that neither could produce alone. Drugs that work together are said to be synergistic.

Potentiation. The action of two drugs in which one prolongs or multiplies the effect of the other. Drug A may be said to potentiate the effect of drug B.

Antagonism. The opposing action of two drugs in which one decreases or cancels out the effect of the other. Drug A may be referred to as an antagonist of drug B.

It is extremely important for the prescribing physician to know of all medications that a patient is taking in order to prevent undesirable drug interactions. On the other hand, it may be intentionally ordered that two drugs be taken together, because some drug interactions are desirable and beneficial. Compare the following situations, describing both desirable and undesirable drug interactions:

Desirable synergism. Promethazine (Phenergan) (a nonnarcotic sedative) and meperidine (Demerol) (a narcotic analgesic) are very effective in relieving pain. By giving small amounts of each together, pain can be relieved more safely than by giving a large amount of Demerol (which is addictive) by itself.

Undesirable synergism. Sedatives and barbiturates given in combination can depress the central nervous system (CNS) to dangerous levels, depending on the strengths of each.

Desirable potentiation. To build up a high level of some forms of penicillin (an antibiotic) in the blood, the drug probenecid (Benemid) (antigout medication) can be given simultaneously. Benemid potentiates the effect of penicillin by slowing the excretion rate of the antibiotic.

Undesirable potentiation. Toxic effects may result when cimetidine (Tagamet) (a gastric antisecretory) is given simultaneously with Tofranil (an antidepressant). Tagamet potentiates the level of antidepressant concentrations in the blood.

Desirable antagonism. A narcotic antagonist (e.g., naloxone, Narcan) saves lives from drug overdoses by canceling out the effect of narcotics.

Undesirable antagonism. Antacids taken at the same time as tetracycline alter the pH and prevent absorption of tetracycline.

DOSAGE

Different dosages of a drug may bring about variations in the speed of drug action or effectiveness. *Dosage* is defined as that amount of drug that is given for a particular therapeutic or desired effect. Terms for various dosage levels are:

1. *Minimum dose.* Smallest amount of a drug that will produce a therapeutic effect
2. *Maximum dose.* Largest amount of a drug that will produce a desired effect without producing symptoms of toxicity
3. *Loading dose.* Initial high dose (often maximum dose) used to quickly elevate the level of the drug in the blood (often followed by a series of lower maintenance doses)
4. *Maintenance dose.* Dose required to keep the drug blood level at a steady state in order to maintain the desired effect
5. *Toxic dose.* Amount of a drug that will produce harmful side effects or symptoms of poisoning
6. *Lethal dose.* Dose that is fatal or causes death
7. *Usual dose.* Dose that is customarily given (average adult dose based on body weight of 150 lb); adjusted according to variations from the norm

You may be familiar with the use of a high loading dose followed by a lesser maintenance dose. If you have taken antibiotics, you may have been instructed to take two tablets or capsules initially and then take one tablet every six hours. It is frequently desirable to give a loading dose of antibiotics to build up a high level and get the process of killing the bacteria started.

ROUTE

The route of administration is probably the most significant factor in the speed of drug action.

The route of drug administration can be compared to the route of travel. In planning a trip from point A to point B, you may have a map that shows several courses of travel to reach the destination. The course you select is optional, depending on your choice for the quickest, cheapest, safest, or most scenic route.

Options for routes of drug administration are much the same. There are a number of methods by which drugs may be given to reach their destination. Sometimes the route selected is based on the degree of speed, cost, or safety of administration. Sometimes there is no choice of routes because some medications can be given only by one route. Often this is because absorption occurs by that route only, or the substance is dangerous or toxic when given by another route. Insulin, for example, may be given only by injection. Much research has been done to produce an oral form of insulin, but attempts have failed because the drug is destroyed by gastric juices.

The most common routes of administration may be grouped into two main categories:

1. GI tract routes
   a. Oral (PO)
   b. Nasogastric tube
   c. Rectal (R)
2. Parenteral routes, which include any other than the gastrointestinal tract
   a. Sublingual (SL) or buccal
   b. Injection routes
      i. Intraveneous (IV)
      ii. Intramuscular (IM)
      iii. Subcutaneous (SC)
      iv. Intradermal (ID)
      v. Intracardiac, Intraspinal, Intracapsular*
   c. Topical (T)
      i. Dermal (D)
      ii. Mucosal
   d. Inhalation

There are advantages and disadvantages in the use of each route. The doctor's choice of a particular route of administration of a drug may depend on (1) desired effects (e.g., fast or slow, local or systemic); (2) absorption qualities of the drug; and (3) how the drug is supplied. Other general points regarding the effect of the route on the drug absorption are as follows:

1. The oral route is the easiest, but the effects are slower because of the time required for disintegration of drugs in the alimentary canal before absorption.
2. The intravenous route is the *fastest* (Fig. 3.4). Drugs enter the bloodstream immediately. Doses to be given IV are in small amounts; effects are immediate and can be quite dangerous if given in amounts recommended for other routes.
   a. IVs are administered by a physician, registered nurse, or paramedic.
   b. IV is the best route for treatment of emergencies because of the speed of action.
3. Parenteral routes are the choice when:
   a. Patient can take nothing by mouth (NPO).

*The latter three injection routes are less common.

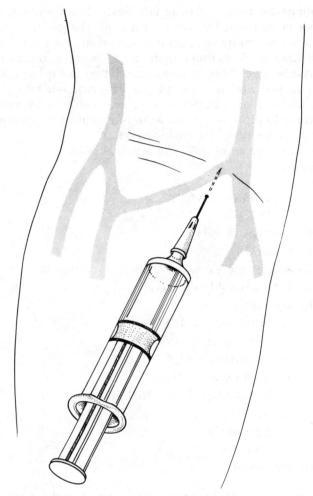

Figure 3.4 *Intravenous route. The IV route is the fastest. Drugs given intravenously enter the bloodstream immediately, since no time is required for absorption.*

    b. The drug is not suitable for GI absorption.

4. The intramuscular route is fairly rapid because the muscles are highly vascular. If it is desirable to retard the speed of absorption, a drug to be given IM may be added to an oily base.

Unexpected Responses to Drugs

Several other terms must be defined in order to complete your awareness of the bodily effects of drugs. These terms refer to adverse drug effects.

Teratogenic effect. Effect from maternal drug administration that causes the development of physical defects in a fetus.

Idiosyncracy. Unique, unusual response to a drug. For example, a patient may have an idiosyncracy to a particular tranquilizer if it causes agitation and excitement rather than tranquility.

Tolerance. Decreased response to a drug that develops after repeated doses are given. To achieve the desired effect, the drug dosage must be increased or the drug replaced.

Dependence. Acquired need for a drug that may produce psychological and/or physical symptoms of withdrawal when the drug is discontinued.

- Psychological dependence involves only a psychological craving; no physical symptoms of withdrawal other than anxiety.
- Physical dependence exists when cells actually have a need for the drug; symptoms of withdrawal include retching, nausea, pain, tremors, and sweating.

Hypersensitivity. Immune response (allergy) to a drug may be of varying degrees.

- May be mild with no immediate effects; rash may appear after 3–4 days of drug therapy.
- May develop after uneventful previous uses of a drug.
- More likely to exist in patients with other known allergies.

Extreme caution should be taken when giving a new medication to a patient for the first time, particularly if the patient has a history of other allergies.

Anaphylactic reaction. Severe, possibly fatal, allergic (hypersensitivity) response.

- Signs include itching, urticaria (hives), hyperemia (reddened, warm skin), vascular collapse, shock, cyanosis, laryngeal edema, and dyspnea.
- Treatment includes cardiopulmonary resuscitation (CPR) if indicated and drugs as required: epinephrine (Adrenalin) to raise blood pressure; corticosteroid (Solu-Medrol) to reduce inflammation and the body's immunological response, antihistamine (Benadryl) to suppress histamine, thereby reducing redness, itching, and edema.
- Anaphylaxis has been noted often with the following: antibiotics, especially penicillin; X-ray dyes containing iodides (IVP dye, angiogram dye; gallbladder dyes; etc.); foods (shellfish, onions, peanuts, etc.); and insect stings (bees and ants).

Knowledge of any adverse reactions to drugs should be included in the patient's history. This information can be helpful in preventing repeated episodes. Getting an accurate drug history and clearly listing known allergies is a critical function of the health care worker.

Persons who have had an anaphylactic reaction to a substance should always wear a Medic-Alert tag or bracelet to identify the substance to which they are extremely allergic. Persons who have had hypersensitivity reactions to a substance are more at risk for reactions to other substances as well.

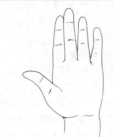

STOP!
Check your knowledge of this chapter before going any further.

CHAPTER REVIEW QUIZ

Fill in the blanks.

1.

Drug Sources	Example	Trade Name	Classification

2. Drugs that are distributed throughout the body have _____ effects.

3. Drugs whose action is limited to a specific location have _____ effects.

4. As drugs pass through the body, they undergo four processes:

Process	Definition of Process

5. Factors that may affect the passage of drugs through the body:

Process	Primary Site of Process	Conditions Hampering Process

6. If circulation is poor, metabolism faulty, or excretion inadequate, drugs may build up in the system, leading to _____ effects, causing poisonous, or _____ , levels of the drug.

7. Variables affecting the efficiency of drug action include _____ , _____ , _____ , and _____ .

Match the term with the definition:

8. Synergism _____   a. Amount of drug required to keep drug level steady

9. Antagonism _____   b. Amount of drug that can cause death

10. Potentiation _____   c. Amount of drug that can cause dangerous side effects

11. Lethal dose _____   d. One drug making the effect of another drug more powerful

12. Toxic dose _____   e. Drugs working together for a better effect

13. Maintenance dose _____   f. Drugs working against each other or counteracting each other's effect

14. Idiosyncracy _____   a. Acquired need for a drug, with symptoms of withdrawal when discontinued

15. Tolerance _____   b. Unusual response to a drug, other than expected effect

16. Dependence _____   c. Effects on a fetus from maternal use of a drug

17. Teratogenic _____   d. Decreased response after repeated use of a drug, increased dosage required for effect

Fill in the blanks:

18. An allergy or immune response to a drug is called _____ .

19. Allergic reactions to drugs may be *mild*, with symptoms such as _____ .

20. Allergic reactions to drugs are more common in patients with _____ .

21. *Severe* allergic reaction with shock, laryngeal edema, and dyspnea is called _____ .

22. Treatment of severe allergic reactions include the following three medications in order of administration: _____ , _____ , and _____ .

4

Medication Preparations and Supplies

OBJECTIVES

Upon completion of this chapter, the student will be able to:

1. Differentiate between various oral drug forms: sublingual tablet versus buccal tablet, solution versus suspension, syrup versus elixir, enteric-coated tablet versus scored tablet, and timed-release capsule versus lozenge.
2. Explain what is meant by parenteral.
3. Give four classifications of drugs that are commonly given by the rectal route.
4. Define the following types of injections and explain how they differ in administration and absorption rate: IV, IM, SC, and ID.
5. Compare the IV injections referred to as IV push, IV infusion, and IV piggyback.
6. List and define at least eight drug forms used for topical (both dermal and mucosal) administration.
7. Explain the advantages of administering drugs via a dermal patch.
8. Identify various supplies used in the preparation of medications.

The forms in which drugs are prepared are as numerous as the routes of administration. *Drug form* refers to the type of preparation in which the drug is supplied. Pharmaceutical companies prepare each drug in the form or forms most suitable for its intended route and means of absorption. *Drug form* and *drug preparation* are synonymous. The *PDR* lists the forms available for each drug under the heading "How Supplied." See Table 4.1 for abbreviations of some of the drug forms and routes of administration.

TABLE 4.1. ABBREVIATIONS FOR DRUG ADMINISTRATION

Drug Forms			Routes
cap	capsule	D	dermal
elix	elixir	ID	intradermal
		IM	intramuscular
gtt	drops	IV	intravenous
supp	suppository	IVPB	intravenous piggyback
susp	suspension	PO, p.o., per os	oral
tab	tablet	R	rectal
ung	ointment	SC, subcu, subq	subcutaneous
		T	topical

A Space-Age Drug Form

Great advances have occurred recently in developing a new drug form that may revolutionize the way a number of drugs are administered. The new drug form is the dermal patch, or *transdermal delivery system*. Dermal patches have been taken on the space shuttles during the 1980s for the prevention of nausea. The key to the transdermal system is that the drug molecules are present in a variety of sizes and shapes that allow for absorption through the skin at various rates. Thus, a patch can provide a constant, even flow of a drug over a long period of time — hours or days. The drug, being released at a consistent rate, remains at an effective level in the blood, as opposed to rising and falling, as happens with pills. Advantages of this method of administration include:

- Easy application, with no discomfort or undesirable taste
- Effectiveness for long periods of time, hours for some drugs and days for others
- Consistent blood level of drug, since drug is released at varying rates, rather than all at one time

Dermal patches vary in size, shape, and color (Fig. 4.1). They are most commonly seen today on patients for the prevention of angina. Current marketing of dermal patches includes those for the prevention of motion sickness (may be applied before traveling) as well as those for the prevention of angina (nitro-

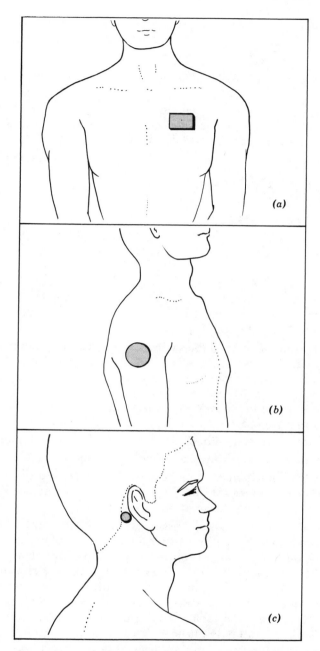

Figure 4.1 *Transdermal drug delivery. Dermal patches vary in size, shape, and color. (a, b) For prevention of angina pectoris; (c) for prevention of motion sickness.*

glycerin). Research is ongoing in the development of dermal patches for birth control, cancer, high blood pressure, ulcers, allergies, and heart conditions. Probably not all drug molecules will be adaptable to this drug form, but it certainly has opened new doors in the area of drug administration.

Standard Drug Forms

You probably have received medications in many of the standard forms at some time during your life. Each form is defined and listed below according to the routes of administration (see Fig. 4.2). As you read in Chapter 3, drugs may be administered through the GI tract or parenterally. GI routes include oral, nasogastric tube, and rectal. Parenteral refers to any route not involving the GI tract, including injection, topical (skin or mucosal), and inhalation routes.

ORAL DRUG FORMS

Oral drug forms include:

Tablet. Disk of compressed drug; may be a variety of shapes and colors; may be coated to enhance easy swallowing; may be *scored* (evenly divided in halves or quarters by score lines) to enhance equal distribution of drug if it has been broken.

Enteric-coated tablet. Tablet with a special coating that resists disintegration by gastric juices. The coating dissolves further down the GI tract, in the enteric, or intestinal, region. Some drugs, such as aspirin, that are irritating to the stomach are available in enteric-coated tablets. To be effective, the coating must never be destroyed by chewing or crushing when it is administered.

Capsule. Drug contained within a gelatin-type container.
- Easier to swallow than noncoated tablets.
- Double chamber may be pulled apart to add drug powder to soft foods or beverages for patients who have difficulty swallowing (unless specifically contraindicated for absorption).

Timed-release (sustained-release) capsule. Capsule containing drug particles that have various coatings (often of different colors) that differ in the amount of time required before the coatings dissolve. This form of drug preparation is designed to deliver a dose of drug over an extended period of time. An advantage of taking a drug in the timed-release form is the decreased frequency of administration. For example, the tranquilizer Valium may be administered in tablet form, 5 mg tid or in the timed-release form (Valrelease, 15 mg) only once qd. Because of the significance of the various coatings that encapsulate the drug particles, it is important that the small colored pellets *not* be crushed or mixed with foods. Damage to the coatings of drug pellets allow the drug to be released all at one time as it is administered. Such immediate release of drug is a potential overdose. Timed-release capsules should be swallowed whole, with no physical damage to the contents of the capsule.

Lozenge (troche). Tablet containing palatable flavoring, indicated for a local (often soothing) effect on the throat or mouth.
- Patient is advised *not* to swallow a lozenge; it should be allowed to slowly dissolve in the mouth.

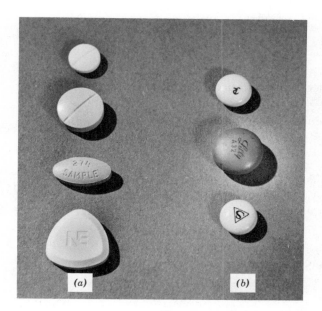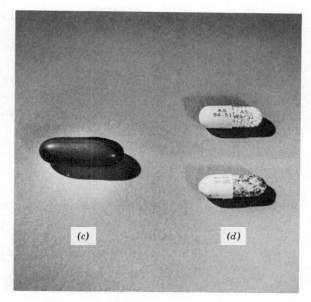

Figure 4.2 *Oral drug forms. Tablets and capsules vary in size, shape, and color.* (a) *Tablets, scored and unscored;* (b) *enteric-coated tablets;* (c) *gelatin capsule;* (d) *timed-release capsules.*

- Patient is also advised not to drink liquids for approximately 15 min after administration, to prevent washing of the lozenge contents from the throat or mouth.

Suspension. Liquid form of medication that must be shaken well before administration because the drug particles settle at the bottom of the bottle. The drug is not evenly dissolved in the liquid.

- A cephalosporin, (Keflex) suspension is a commonly used antibiotic suspension for children. This form is more easily ingested by children than are capsules of Keflex.

Emulsion. Liquid drug preparation that contains oils and fats in water.

Elixir, fluid extract. Liquid drug forms with alcohol base.

- Should be tightly capped to prevent alcohol evaporation.
- Should not be available to alcoholics.

Syrup. Sweetened, flavored liquid drug form. Cherry syrup drug preparations are common for children.

Solution. Liquid drug form in which the drug is totally evenly dissolved. Appearance is clear, rather than cloudy or settled (as with a suspension).

The drug forms for the oral route are commonly available over the counter and include thousands of trade name products. The oral route is the easiest and probably the cheapest for administration. It is, however, *not* the route of choice for treatment of emergencies, acute pain, NPO patients, or patients unable to swallow. Other routes, especially the parenteral routes, produce a more rapid absorption rate and drug effect.

RECTAL DRUG FORMS

Rectal drug forms include:

Suppository. Drug suspended in a substance, such as cocoa butter, that melts at body temperature.

Enema solution. Drug suspended in solution to be administered as an enema.

The rectal route of administration is often the choice if the patient is ordered to have NPO or cannot swallow. The most common classifications of drugs given rectally include sedatives, antiemetics, and antipyretics. A local analgesic effect may also be achieved by this route. In the past, rectal administration of drug solutions was given for general anesthesia, but is not common today.

INJECTABLE DRUG FORMS

Injectable drug forms include:

Solution. Drug suspended in a sterile vehicle.
- Quite often the solutions have a sterile water base and are thus referred to as *aqueous* (aq) (waterlike) solutions.
- Some solutions have an oil base, which tends to cause a more prolonged absorption time. The oily nature of these solutions makes them thick; thus they are referred to as *viscous* (thick) solutions.

Powder. Dry particles of drugs. The powder itself cannot be injected. It must be mixed with a sterile diluting solution (sterile water or saline solution) to render an injectable solution. This is termed *reconstitution* of a drug. Drugs are supplied undiluted in powder form because of the short period of time they remain stable after dilution.

The various injection routes differ according to the type of tissues into which the drug is deposited and the rate of absorption. Each is briefly defined below:

Intravenous. Injected directly into a vein. Immediate absorption and availability to major organs renders this route too dangerous for administration by those other than physicians, paramedics, or registered nurses. Types of intravenous injections include:
- IV push (IVP), a small volume of drug injected through a syringe into the bloodstream.
- IV infusion or IV drip, a large volume of fluids, often with drugs added, which infuses continually into a vein.
- IV piggyback (IVPB), a drug diluted in moderate volume (50–100 ml) of fluid for intermittent infusion at specified intervals, usually q6–8h; the diluted solution is infused (piggyback) into a port on the main IV tubing or into a rubber adapter on the IV catheter (Fig. 4.3).

Intramuscular. Injected into a muscle, by positioning the needle and syringe at a 90-degree angle from the skin (Fig. 4.4). Absorption is fairly rapid due to the vascularity of muscle.

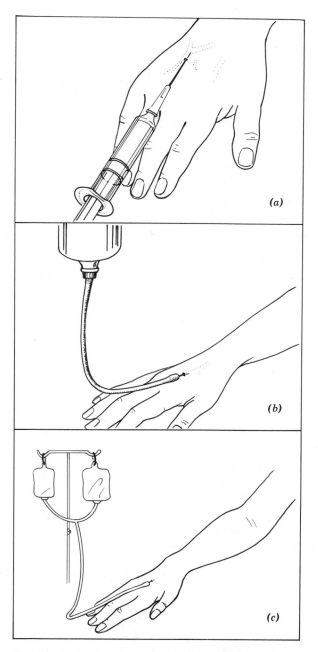

Figure 4.3 *Intravenous administration. Different forms of IV injection include* (a) *IV push;* (b) *IV infusion (continuous); and* (c) *IV piggyback (intermittent).*

Subcutaneous. Injected into the fatty layer of tissue below the skin by positioning the needle and syringe at a 45-degree angle from the skin (Fig. 4.5). This may be the route of choice for drugs that should not be absorbed as rapidly as through the IV or IM routes.

Intradermal. Injected just beneath the skin, by positioning the needle and sy-

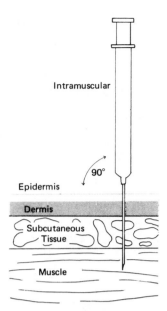

Figure 4.4 *Intramuscular injection. Needle is inserted at a 90-degree angle.*

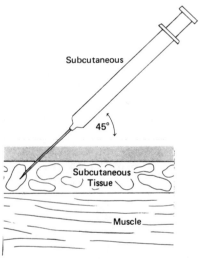

Figure 4.5 *Subcutaneous injection. Needle is inserted at a 45-degree angle.*

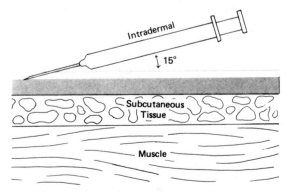

Figure 4.6 *Intradermal injection. Needle is inserted just beneath the skin at a 15-degree angle.*

ringe at a 15-degree angle from the skin (Fig. 4.6). This route is used primarily for allergy skin testing. Because of the lack of vascularity in the dermis, absorption is slow. The greatest reaction is in the local tissues rather than systemic. When a small amount (0.1–0.2 cc) of drug is injected intradermally, the amount of redness that develops around the injection site can be used to determine whether a person is sensitive to the drug. A positive reaction to a foreign bacteria, as in a tuberculin (TB) skin test, (PPD) may indicate that the individual does not have sufficient antibodies against the disease-producing bacteria.

The less common parenteral routes, which are limited to a physician's administration, are:

Intracardiac. Injected directly into the heart. This route is used to administer adrenalin as a last resort to resuscitate a patient whose heart has stopped.

Intraspinal. Injected into the subarachnoid space, which contains cerebrospinal fluid (CSF) and surrounds the spinal cord. Drugs injected by this route are anesthetics, which render a lack of sensation to those regions of the body distal to the intraspinal injection.

Intracapsular (intraarticular). Injected into the capsule of a joint, usually to reduce inflammation, as in bursitis. Arthritic or bursitic joints often injected with anti-inflammatory drugs include shoulders, elbows, wrists, ankles, knees, and hips.

TOPICAL DRUG FORMS

Topical drug forms include drugs for dermal application and drugs for mucosal application. Those for *dermal* application include:

Cream ointment. A semisolid preparation containing a drug, for external application.

Lotion. A liquid preparation applied externally for treatment of skin disorders. Unlike hand lotions, medicated lotions (e.g., calamine lotion) should be *patted,* not rubbed, on the affected skin.

Liniment. Preparation for external use that is rubbed on the skin as a counterirritant. As such, the liniment creates a different sensation (e.g., tingling or burning) to mask pain in the skin or muscles.

Dermal patch. Skin patch containing drug molecules that can be absorbed through the skin at varying rates to promote a consistent blood level between application times.

Both the dermal patch and ointment are common forms for administration of nitroglycerin. Nitroglycerin is a vasodilator used for the treatment of angina (chest pain related to narrowing of the coronary arteries). The beauty of the external applications of nitroglycerin is their ability to *prevent* angina by the slow, consistent release of the drug over a period of time. Before the external applications became available, nitroglycerin was primarily available in the form of a sublingual tablet to be taken at the time of an angina attack. Now all three forms are used — the tablet, the ointment, and the patch — with the external forms

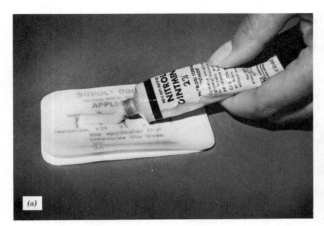
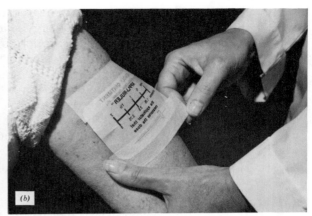

Figure 4.7   *Topical administration. Dermal application includes creams, ointments, and liquids placed on the skin. (a) Nitroglycerin ointment is measured on Appli-Ruler paper. (b) Paper containing ointment is applied to the skin.*

focusing on the prevention of angina. They are applied at regular intervals, as follows:

> *Ointment:* 1–5 inches applied q8h measured and applied on special Appliruler paper (Fig. 4.7)
>
> *Dermal patch:* one patch (available in varied doses) q24h

Other drug preparations considered topical are those that are applied to *mucosal membranes.* Some are administered for local effect (at the site of application) and, in other cases, a systemic effect is desired. The *mucosal drug forms* include:

> *Eye, ear, and nose drops (gtt).* Drugs in sterile liquids to be applied by drops (referred to as *instillation* of drops).
>
> *Eye ointment.* Sterile semisolid preparation, often antibiotic in nature, for ophthalmic use only.
>
> *Vaginal creams.* Medicated creams, often of antibiotic or antifungal nature, that are to be inserted vaginally with the use of a special applicator.
>
> *Rectal and vaginal suppositories.* Drug suspended in a substance, such as cocoa butter, that melts at body temperature, for local effect. Some rectal suppositories are also used for systemic effects (Fig. 4.8).
>
> *Douche solution.* Sterile solution, often an antiseptic such as povidone iodine solution and sterile water, used to irrigate the vaginal canal.
>
> *Buccal tablet.* Tablet that is absorbed *via the buccal mucosa* in the mouth.
> - Patient is told *not* to swallow tablet; it is to be placed between the cheek and gums, and allowed to dissolve slowly.
> - Not commonly used today.
>
> *Sublingual tablet.* Tablet that is absorbed *via the mucosa* under the tongue.
> - Patient is told *not* to swallow tablet; it is to be placed under the tongue and allowed to dissolve slowly.
> - The most common sublingual tablet is nitroglycerin. Given for the treatment of angina, this drug reaches the bloodstream immediately via the sublingual capillaries. Angina may be relieved within 1–5 min after sublingual nitroglycerin is administered.

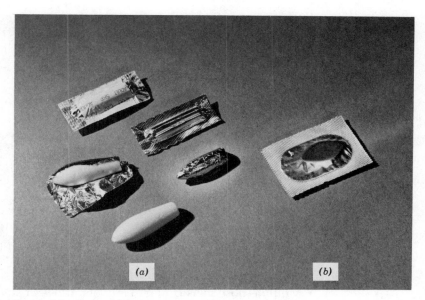

Figure 4.8 *Topical administration via mucous membranes. Suppositories come in various shapes and sizes, for example, (a) rectal suppositories, wrapped in foil and unwrapped; and (b) vaginal suppository, wrapped in foil.*

INHALABLE DRUG FORMS

The drug forms used for the inhalation route include:

Spray or mist. Liquid drug forms that may be inhaled as fine droplets via the use of spray bottles or nebulizers.
- In the hospital setting, respiratory therapists instill a liquid into a chamber of a nebulizer for a patient's breathing treatment. Often the liquid contains a bronchodilator, a mucolytic agent, or sterile saline solution for moisture.
- In the home, the patient may instill sprays via nasal spray bottles, vaporizers, or inhalers. Asthma patients rely on the use of inhalers to keep their bronchioles open by inhaling the mist of a bronchodilator. A mouthpiece, through which the patient inhales, is connected to a bottle of liquid drug.

Gas. Anesthetics, such as nitrous oxide, that are introduced via the respiratory route for general anesthesia.

Powder. Drug in powder form for relief of bronchial asthma, to be inhaled through a special device called a spinhaler. The powdered drug, cromolyn sodium, (Intal) is inside a capsule that is inserted into the spinhaler.

Supplies

Considering the variety of drug forms you may be administering, you must become familiar with various supplies to be used (Fig. 4.9):

Medicine cup. Two types of disposable cups are commonly used. Paper cups are used for dispensing tablets and capsules. Plastic 1-oz medicine cups with measurements (ml, tsp, tbsp, dr, or oz) marked on the side, are used for dispensing oral liquid medications and tablets or capsules. (See Table 5.1 for a list of common abbreviations used in medication orders.)

Mortar. Glass cup in which tablets (excluding enteric-coated tablets) may be placed to be crushed.

Pestle. Club-shaped glass tool used as the crushing device to pulverize tablets.

Finger cot. Rubber coverlet for one finger only, to be applied and lubricated before insertion of a rectal suppository (Fig. 4.10).

Medication for injection is contained in ampule or vial (Fig. 4.11):

Ampule. Small glass container that holds a single dose of sterile solution for injection. The ampule must be broken at the neck to obtain the solution.

Vial. Glass container sealed at the top by a rubber stopper to enhance sterility of the contents. Contents may be a solution or a powdered drug that needs to be reconstituted. Vials may be multiple dose or unit dose:

- Multiple-dose vials contain large quantities of solution (up to 50 cc) and may repeatedly be entered through the rubber stopper to remove a portion of the contents.
- Unit-dose vials contain small quantities of solution (1–2 cc) that are removed during a single use. Unit-dose vials are widely used today as a means of controlling abuse or removal of excess amounts of solution from a drug vial.

Needles. Needles for injections have two measurements that must be noted (Fig. 4.12):

- Length varies from short (⅜ inch) to medium (1½ inch) length for standard injections. Long needles (5 inch) may be used by the physician for intraspinal or intracardiac routes.
- Gauge is a number that represents the diameter of the needle lumen. Needle gauges vary from 18 (largest) to 27 (smallest), with the higher gauge number representing the smaller lumen.

Syringes. The three most common disposable syringes for parenteral administration of drugs are the standard hypodermic syringe, the tuberculin (TB) syringe, and the insulin syringe (Fig. 4.13).

- The standard hypodermic syringe has a capacity of 2½–3 cc. Most companies prepackage this type of syringe with a needle attached. Since you may use this type of syringe for either subcutaneous or intramuscular injections, you must choose the package with the needle length and gauge appropriate for the route and depth of injection you will give. All hypodermic syringes are marked with 10 calibrations per cc. Thus, each small line represents 0.1 cc. When preparing for an injection with this syringe, you must know the amount of solution needed to the nearest 0.1 cc (an additional scale on the syringe shows calibrations in minims, which is discussed later, in Chapter 9.)
- The TB syringe is very narrow and is finely calibrated. The total capacity is only 1 cc. There are 100 fine calibration lines marking the capacity. Thus, each line represents 0.01 cc. Every tenth line is longer, to indicate 0.1-cc increments. Very precise small amounts of solution may be mea-

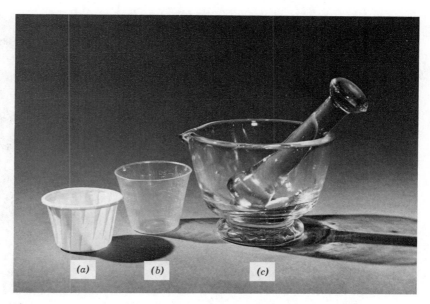

Figure 4.9 *Supplies for oral administration. (a) Tablets and capsules are usually administered in paper soufflé cups. (b) Liquids are measured in calibrated plastic cups. (c) A mortar and pestle are used when necessary to crush tablets.*

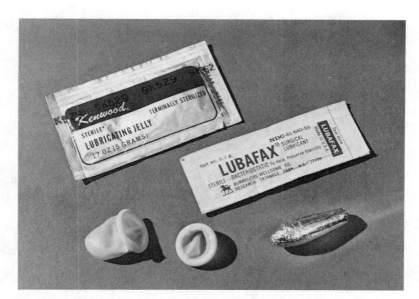

Figure 4.10 *Supplies for administration of a rectal suppository. A finger cot and small packet of lubricant are required.*

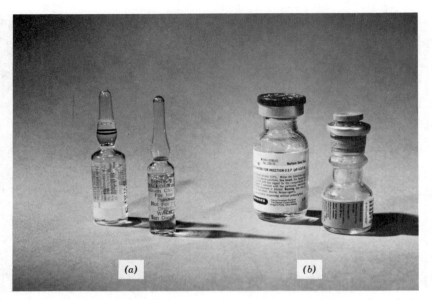

Figure 4.11 *Medication for injection. Various premeasured containers include* (a) *ampules and* (b) *vials.*

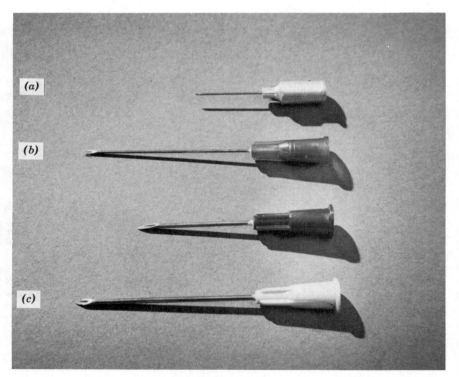

Figure 4.12 *Needles commonly used for injections. Sizes vary in length and gauge.* (a) ³⁄₈ *inch, 27 gauge;* (b) *1½ inches, 21 gauge;* (c) *1 inch and 1½ inches, 18 gauge.*

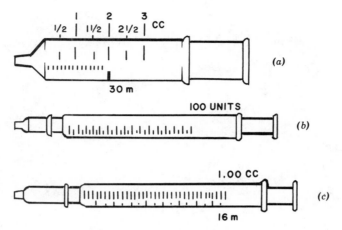

Figure 4.13 *Syringes for injection. Type of syringe varies with type and quantity of medication. (a) Standard 3-ml hypodermic syringe; (b) insulin syringe; (c) tuberculin syringe.*

sured with the TB syringe. It is most commonly used for newborn and pediatric dosages and for intradermal skin tests. When preparing for an injection with this syringe, you must know the amount of solution needed to the nearest 0.01 cc.

The insulin syringe is used strictly for administrating insulin to diabetics. Like the TB syringe, it has only a 1-cc capacity. The 1 cc capacity is marked as 100 units (U) to represent a strength of 100 U of insulin when full. Each group of 10 U is further divided by 5 small lines on an even scale or 5 small lines on an odd scale. Thus, each line represents 2 U. A smaller insulin syringe, of only ½ cc capacity, may be used when less than 50 U (½ cc) of insulin is ordered. The smaller insulin syringe has 50 small calibration lines; thus, each represents 1 U of insulin.

It is extremely important that you can interpret the value of the calibrations on each of the syringes. Study the calibrations each time you prepare for an injection to prevent a medication error from negligent misinterpretation.

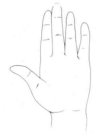

STOP!
Check your knowledge of this chapter before going any further.

CHAPTER REVIEW QUIZ

1. Which route of administration is used most often? Why?

    _____

    _____

Complete with the appropriate drug form:

2. A tablet placed under the tongue: _____

3. A tablet placed in the cheek pouch: _____

4. A tablet dissolved in the mouth for local action: _____

5. A coated tablet that dissolves in the intestines instead of in the stomach:

    _____

6. A capsule that has delayed action over a longer period of time:

    _____

7. A liquid drug form with an alcohol base: _____

8. A liquid medication that must be shaken before administration:

    _____

9. Drugs given by the rectal route include _____

    and _____ .

10. The parenteral route refers to any route other than the gastrointestinal route. Name four parenteral routes:

    _____

    _____

    _____

    _____

Fill in the blanks:

11. Crushing tablets requires a _____ and _____ .

12. To administer a rectal suppository, you need a _____ and

    _____ .

13. Medicine for injection is contained in two types of glass containers:

    a. With rubber stopper on top: _____

    b. All glass to be broken at the neck: _____

14. Needles are selected according to two measurements: _____ and _____ .

15. The three most commonly used syringes for injections are: _____ , _____ , and _____ .

5

Abbreviations and Systems of Measurement

OBJECTIVES

Upon completion of this chapter, the student will be able to:

1. Identify common abbreviations and symbols used for medication orders.
2. List the six parts of a medication order and the two additional items required on a prescription blank.
3. Describe the responsibilities of the health care worker regarding verbal and telephone orders for medications.
4. Interpret medication orders correctly.
5. Compare and contrast the three systems of measurement.
6. Convert dosages from one system to another by use of the table for metric, apothecary, and household equivalents.
7. Describe appropriate patient education for those who will be measuring and administering their own medications.

Abbreviations

Interpretation of the medication order is the first responsibility when preparing medication for administration. Knowledge of abbreviations and symbols is essential for accurate interpretation of the physician's order. The abbreviations and symbols in Table 5.1 must be memorized. You may see some abbreviations written with or without periods, and orders may vary in the use of capital versus lowercase letters. You may occasionally see other abbreviations not included in this list. When in doubt, always question the meaning.

Medication orders contain six parts:

1. Date.
2. Patient's name.
3. Medication name.
4. Dosage or amount of medication.
5. Route or manner of administration (if no route is specified, the oral route is assumed).
6. Time to be administered or frequency.

Medication orders must always be written and signed by a physician. In an emergency the physician may give a verbal order. It is the responsibility of the health care worker to repeat the order (i.e., medication and amount) before administration and to write down medication, amount, and time of administration as soon as it is given. The physician will sign the medication order after the emergency. Always determine the policy of the agency before taking a telephone order. Most agencies require a registered nurse to take telephone orders, and the order must be signed by the physician within 24 hours.

Medication orders can be written on the patient's record in the physician's office, clinic, or institution, or on a prescription blank (Fig. 5.1). It is the responsibility of the health care worker to check the medication order for completeness by noting the six items — date, patient name, medication name, dosage, route, and frequency (plus additional items if using the prescription blank) — and to question any discrepancy, omission, or unusual order. The prescription blank contains two additional items: the physician's Drug Enforcement Administration registration number) if the medication is a controlled substance and the number of times that the prescription can be refilled.

Systems of Measurement

In order to carry out a medication order accurately, the person administering medications must have an understanding of the different systems of measurement. The original system of weights and measures for writing medication orders was the *apothecary system.* An apothecary is a pharmacist or druggist. Some physicians still order drugs by the apothecary system. However, the *metric system* is the preferred system of measurement and is used more frequently at the present time. The third system of measurement is the *household system,* which is

TABLE 5.1. COMMON ABBREVIATIONS FOR MEDICATION ORDERS

aa, $\overline{aa}$	of each	NS, N/S	normal saline (sodium chloride, 0.9%)
ac	before meals	OD	right eye; overdose
ad lib	as desired	OS	left eye
AM, am	morning	os	mouth
amp	ampule	OU	both eyes
amt	amount	oz, $\overline{3}$	ounce
aq	water	pc	after meals
bid	twice a day	per	by means of
$\overline{c}$	with	PM, pm	afternoon
cap	capsule	po, PO, per os	by mouth, orally
cc	cubic centimeter (equivalent to ml)	PRN, prn	whenever necessary
DC, disc	discontinue	pt	pint
dr, $\overline{3}$	dram	$\overline{q}$	every
D/RL	dextrose $\overline{c}$ Ringer's lactate solution	qd	every day
		qh	every hour
DW	distilled water	q2h	every 2 hours
D₅W	dextrose, 5% in water	q3h	every 3 hours
elix	elixir	qid	four times a day
et	and	qod	every other day
ext	extract	qs	quantity sufficient
fl, fld	fluid	qt	quart
g, Gm	gram	R	rectal
gr	grain	RL, R/L	Ringer's lactate
gtt	drops	Rx	take
h, hr	hour	$\overline{s}$	without
H	hypodermic	SC, subcu, subq	subcutaneous
hs, HS	at bedtime, at hour of sleep	sig	label
IM	intramuscular	SL	sublingual
IV	intravenous	sol	solution
IVP	intravenous push or intravenous pyelogram	sos	once if necessary
		sp	spirits
IVPB	intravenous piggyback	ss, $\overline{ss}$	one-half
kg, Kg	kilogram	stat	immediately
KVO, TKO	keep vein open, to keep open	supp	suppository
L	liter	syr	syrup
lb	pound	T	temperature
m, ɱ, min	minim	tab	tablet
mEq	milliequivalent	tbsp, T, tbs	tablespoon
μg, mcg	microgram	tid	three times a day
mg	milligram	tinct, tr	tincture
ml	milliliter (equivalent to cc)	tsp, t	teaspoon
NaCl	sodium chloride	U, u	unit
noc, noct, n	night	ung	ointment
NPO, npo	nothing by mouth		

PHONE 366-0000
366-0000

DEA #012345

JACK C. DOE, M.D.
000 DOCTORS PARK
1 MAIN STREET
SARASOTA, FLORIDA 07728

R

SUBSTITUTION ALLOWED _____

PRIOR APPROVAL REQUIRED _____

REFILL: _____   _____ LABEL

Figure 5.1 Prescription blank. Check for completeness and accuracy, including date, patient's name, medication name, dosage, route, frequency or time, number of refills, and DEA number for controlled substances.

the least accurate. However, this system is more familiar to the layperson and is therefore used in prescribing medications for the patient at home. The health care worker must understand all three systems of measurement for accurate administration of medicines and for patient education as well. Medication orders are concerned with only two types of measurement: (1) measuring fluids, or liquid measure, and (2) measuring solids, or solid weight.

The apothecary system of liquid measurement includes the minim, fluid dram, fluid ounce, pint, quart, and gallon. The apothecary system for measuring solid weights includes the grain, dram, ounce, and pound (see Table 5.2).

Rules for writing dosages in the apothecary system are as follows:

TABLE 5.2. ABBREVIATIONS AND SYMBOLS FOR THE APOTHECARY SYSTEM

grain	gr
minim[a]	m, m̖, min
drop[a]	gtt
dram	dr, ℈
ounce	oz, ℥
pint	pt
quart	qt

[a]A drop is approximately equivalent to 1 minim of water, but the type of solution may cause variation. When minims are ordered, they should always be measured with a minim glass or in a tuberculin syringe for accuracy. If the order specifies drops, they may be measured with a medicine dropper.

1. Lowercase Roman numerals are used and *follow* the unit of measurement (e.g., gr iv means 4 grains; ℥⁀ means 2 ounces).
2. The symbol ss may be used for one-half (e.g., gr iss means 1½ grains; gr viiss means 7½ grains).
3. All other fractions are written with Arabic numbers and may precede the unit of measurement (e.g., $\frac{1}{150}$ gr or 3¼ gr).

The metric system was invented by the French in the late eighteenth century and is the international standard for weights and measures. The metric system of liquid measurement includes the liter and the milliliter, which is approximately equivalent to the cubic centimeter. The metric system for measuring solid weights includes the gram and the milligram as the measures most commonly used for medication prescriptions.

At times you will find it necessary to convert a dosage from the apothecary system to the metric or household system. It is important to memorize the few basic equivalents most commonly used. Table 5.3 lists commonly used approximate equivalents for liquid measurement. These figures are easily committed to memory. When conversions are necessary in the measurement of solids, you will find it useful to consult Table 5.4 for metric and apothecary equivalents.

Equipment most commonly used for measuring medications includes the medicine cup and various syringes calibrated in milliliters and/or minims.

PATIENT EDUCATION

When explaining dosage preparation, always speak directly to the patient and observe the patient for comprehension. Many elderly patients have difficulty hearing but are reluctant to admit lack of understanding. Ask them to repeat the directions.

Many elderly patients also have vision problems. Be sure the directions for dosage preparation are written clearly. If a family member will be assisting in preparation and administration of medications, include that person in the instruction. Be sure that any measuring equipment to be used is clearly marked.

Measuring spoons and clearly marked measuring cups should be used when available for household measurement. Such calibrated utensils are more accurate than tableware (Fig. 5.2). Teaspoons, tablespoons, teacups, and drinking glasses vary in size and capacity, and therefore measurements are inaccurate with such utensils.

TABLE 5.3. COMMON APPROXIMATE EQUIVALENTS FOR LIQUID MEASUREMENT

Metric	Apothecary	Household
1 ml	15 m	
5 ml	1 dr	1 tsp
15 ml	4 dr	1 tbsp
30 ml	1 oz	2 tbsp
250 ml	8 oz	1 measuring cup (240 ml)
500 ml	1 pt	
1,000 ml	1 qt (32 oz)	

TABLE 5.4. METRIC AND APOTHECARY EQUIVALENTS FOR SOLID MEASUREMENT

Metric		Apothecary
1 g	**1,000 mg**	**gr xv**
0.6 g	600 mg	gr x
0.5 g	**500 mg**	gr viiss
0.3 g	300 mg	gr v
0.2 g	200 mg	gr iii
0.1 g	100 mg	gr iss
0.06 g	**60 mg**	**gr i**
0.05 g	50 mg	gr ¾
0.03 g	**30 mg**	**gr ½** or **gr ss**
0.02 g	20 mg	gr ⅓
0.015 g	15 mg	gr ¼
0.016 g	16 mg	gr ¼
0.010 g	10 mg	gr ⅙
0.008 g	8 mg	gr ⅛
0.006 g	6 mg	gr 1/10
0.005 g	5 mg	gr 1/12
0.003 g	3 mg	gr 1/20
0.002 g	2 mg	gr 1/30
0.001 g	1 mg	gr 1/60
	0.6 mg	gr 1/100
	0.5 mg	gr 1/120
	0.4 mg	gr 1/150
	0.3 mg	gr 1/200

Note: Memorize all equivalents in boldface.

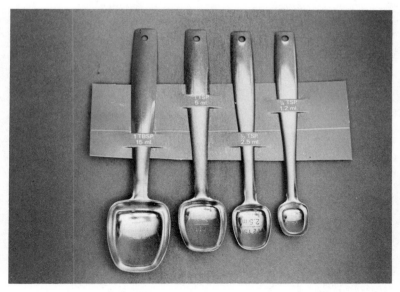

Figure 5.2   *For accurate household measurement, standard measuring spoons are used.*

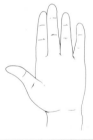

STOP!
Check your knowledge of this chapter before going any further.

CHAPTER REVIEW QUIZ

Interpret the following orders:

1. Keflex 250-mg cap PO q6h

   _____

2. Neosporin ophth sol gtt īī OS qid

   _____

3. Feosol 65 mg tab ī qid pc and hs

   _____

4. Diuril 500 mg PO qAM

   _____

5. Dyazide 1 cap bid

   _____

6. Demerol 50 mg IM q4h prn for pain

   _____

7. Metamucil 1 tsp mixed c̄ 8 ℥ H$_2$O tid ac

   _____

8. Dulcolax supp hs qod prn for constipation

   _____

9. Actifed syr ℥īī qid prn for cough

   _____

10. Nitrostat 1 tab SL prn for angina attack, may repeat q5min ×3

   _____

11. Compazine supp 25 mg sos for nausea

   _____

12. DC Phenergan 48h post-op

   _____

13. Tolinase 250 mg qd c̄ breakfast

   _____

14. Mandol 0.5 g IVPB q8h

   _____

15. Potassium chloride 20 mEq in ½ NS 1L q12h

   _____

16. NPH insulin 20 U SC qd ac breakfast

   _____

17. ASA 5 gr supp R prn T > 101

_____

18. Vasocidin opth sol 1 gtt OD q3h

_____

19. Gargle c̄ ½ peroxide/½ aq sol ad lib s̄ swallowing sol

_____

20. Dalmane 15 mg cap hs prn, may repeat ×1 q noc

_____

Fill in the blanks:

21. Which is the oldest system of measurement for medication?

    _____

22. Which system of drug measurement is used most frequently throughout the world?

    _____

23. Which is the least accurate system for measuring medicine?

    _____

24. Two different types of equipment used to measure drugs are _____ and _____ .

Use Table 5.3 to complete the following conversions, and place the correct answer in the blank:

25. gr V = _____ mg

26. 0.5 mg = gr _____

27. gr × V = _____ g

28. 16 mg = gr _____

29. 1 g = _____ mg

30. gr iss = _____ g

31. gr ⅓ = _____ mg

32. 0.5 g = _____ mg

33. 60 mg = gr _____

34. 1 g = gr _____

35. gr × = _____ mg

36. 1 mg = gr _____

37. 0.1 g = gr _____

38. 0.06 g = gr _____

39. 1 dr = _____ cc = _____ tsp

40. 1 oz = _____ = _____ tbsp

41. 1 cc = _____ min

42. 1 oz = _____ dr

6

Safe Dosage Preparation

OBJECTIVES

Upon completion of this chapter, the student will be able to:

1. Identify the three steps for calculation of the dosage ordered when it differs from the dose on hand.
2. Write the formula for each of the two methods of dosage calculation presented in this chapter.
3. Convert from one system of measurement to another using the ratio and proportion method.
4. Solve dosage problems using the basic calculation method.
5. Solve dosage problems using the ratio and proportion method.
6. List the cautions with the basic calculation method.
7. List the cautions with the ratio and proportion method.

It is the responsibility of the health care worker to be absolutely certain that the medication administered is exactly as prescribed by the physician. Many medications are dispensed now by the pharmacist in unit dose form, in which each individual dose of medicine is prepackaged in a separate packet, vial, or prefilled syringe.

Although much of the mixing and measuring of medications is now completed by the pharmacist, the person who is administering medications must understand the preparation of dosages in order to ensure accuracy. On occasion the dosage ordered differs from the dose on hand. Consequently, it may be necessary to calculate the correct dosage. Calculations can be a simple procedure if you follow the necessary steps in sequential order.

A working knowledge of basic arithmetic is required for accurate calculation of drug dosage. In order to understand the calculation of correct dosage, you must evaluate your basic arithmetic skills by completing the following mathematics pretest. After completing the quiz, check your answers. If there is an error, review mathematics for that area until all problems can be solved accurately and easily. A minimum score of 80% is recommended as indicating readiness for dosage calculations. Those not meeting this criterion should seek remedial assistance in review of basics before beginning calculations.

Basic Arithmetic Test

1. $6\frac{1}{4} + 3\frac{2}{3}$ _____
2. $4\frac{2}{3} - 2\frac{1}{2}$ _____
3. $2\frac{2}{3} \times 3\frac{2}{5}$ _____
4. $\frac{2}{5} \div \frac{3}{4}$ _____
5. $2\frac{2}{3} \div 5$ _____
6. Write six and a third as a decimal. _____
7. $6.67 + .065 + 0.3$ _____
8. $10.4 - .037$ _____
9. $.223 \times .67$ _____
10. $46.72 \div 6.4$ _____
11. Write 8% as a fraction and reduce. _____
12. Change $\frac{2}{5}$ to a decimal. _____
13. Write .023 as a percent. _____
14. Express 12% as a decimal. _____
15. Express .4 as a fraction and reduce. _____
16. Change $\frac{3}{5}$ to a percent. _____
17. Change $12\frac{1}{2}$% to a decimal. _____
18. What is 75% of 160? _____
19. What is 9.2% of 250? _____
20. What is $37\frac{1}{2}$% of 192? _____
21. Which fraction is the largest: $\frac{1}{2}$, $\frac{2}{5}$, or $\frac{3}{10}$? _____
22. Which is the largest: $\frac{1}{3}$, .4, or 60%? _____

23. Write the Roman numeral XXV as an Arabic numeral.   _____
24. Write 154 as a Roman numeral.   _____
25. The label on the bottle reads 0.5 g per tablet. The doctor orders 0.25 g. How many tablets should you give?   _____

ANSWERS TO BASIC ARITHMETIC TEST

1. $9\tfrac{11}{12}$
2. $2\tfrac{1}{6}$
3. $9\tfrac{1}{15}$
4. $\tfrac{8}{15}$
5. $\tfrac{8}{15}$
6. 6.333
7. 7.035
8. 10.363
9. .14941
10. 7.3
11. $\tfrac{2}{25}$
12. .4
13. 2.3%
14. .12
15. $\tfrac{2}{5}$
16. 60%
17. .125
18. 120
19. 23
20. 72
21. $\tfrac{1}{2}$
22. 60%
23. 25
24. CLIV
25. $\tfrac{1}{2}$

Calculation Guidelines

Remember, there is no margin of error in administration of medications. It is possible for a small error in arithmetic to seriously harm a patient. A misplaced decimal point could cause a fatality. Safe dosage preparation requires (1) a working knowledge of basic arithmetic and (2) meticulous care with all calculations.

Calculations can be as simple as 1, 2, 3. When the dosage ordered differs from the dosage on hand, the problem can be solved simply by completing three basic steps:

1. Check whether all measures are in the *same system*. Convert if necessary by using Tables 5.3 and 5.4.
2. Write the problem in equation form using the *appropriate formula and labeling all parts*, and complete the necessary calculations.
3. *Check the accuracy* of your answer for reasonableness, and have someone else *verify* your calculations.

There are several different methods of calculating dosage. Either of the methods presented in this book may be used, or both methods may be used to verify accuracy. The two methods presented here are *basic calculation* and *ratio and proportion*. Basic calculation requires only simple arithmetic, while ratio and proportion requires the ability to determine an unknown, X.

Method 1: Basic Calculation

Use the following formula:

$$\frac{\text{Desired dose}}{\text{On-hand dose}} \times \text{quantity of on-hand dose}$$

in short form:

$$\frac{\text{D}}{\text{OH}} \times \text{Q}$$

EXAMPLE 1

The physician orders aspirin gr 10 q4h PRN for fever over 101°. On hand are aspirin gr 5 tabs.

Step 1. Check to see if all measures are in the same system. No conversion is necessary. Both measures are in grains.

Step 2. Use the formula $\frac{\text{D}}{\text{OH}} \times \text{Q}$ and label all parts:

$$\frac{10 \text{ gr}}{5 \text{ gr}} \times 1 \text{ tab} = 10 \div 5 = 2$$

$$2 \times 1 = 2 \text{ tabs}$$

Note: The labels of the desired and on-hand doses must be the same. The label of the answer must be the same as the quantity.

Step 3. Check for reasonableness. A dose of 2 tabs is within normal limits.

If the calculations resulted in an answer such as ¼ tablet or 3 tablets, the answer is not reasonable and the calculations should be rechecked. If calculations are correct after recheck, any unusual dosage should be checked with the person in charge: the pharmacist or the physician. *When in doubt, always question.*

EXAMPLE 2

The order reads Ampicillin 0.5 g. The unit dose packet reads 250 mg/cap.

Step 1. Check to see if all measures are in the same system. Convert grams to milligrams:

$$1 \text{ g} = 1,000 \text{ mg}$$

$$0.5 \text{ g} = 0.5 \times 1,000 = 500 \text{ mg}$$

Step 2. Use the formula $\dfrac{D}{OH} \times Q$ and label all parts:

$$\frac{500 \text{ mg}}{250 \text{ mg}} \times 1 \text{ cap} =$$

Reduce fractions to lowest terms:

$$\frac{500}{250} = 50 \div 25 = 2$$

$$2 \times 1 = 2 \text{ caps}$$

Step 3. Check for reasonableness. A dose of 2 caps is within normal limits.

EXAMPLE 3

The narcotics drawer contains vials of meperidine (Demerol) labeled 75 mg in 1.5 ml. The preoperative order reads 60 mg IM on call.

Step 1. Check to see if all measures are in the same system. No conversion is necessary.

Step 2. Use the formula $\dfrac{D}{OH} \times Q$ and label all parts:

$$\frac{60 \text{ mg}}{75 \text{ mg}} \times 1.5 \text{ ml} =$$

Reduce fractions to lowest terms:

$$\frac{60}{75} = \frac{12}{15} = \frac{4}{5}$$

Convert fractions to decimals:

$$\frac{4}{5} = 5\overline{)4.0}^{\,0.8}$$

Multiply by quantity.

$$0.8 \times 1.5 \text{ ml} = 1.2 \text{ ml}$$

Note: Fractions must be converted to decimals and rounded off to one decimal place to coincide with the markings on the syringe.

Step 3. Check for reasonableness. A dose of 1.2 ml is within normal limits.

EXAMPLE 4

The physician orders morphine gr ¼ q4h PRN for pain. On hand are vials labeled gr ½ = 1 ml.

Step 1. Check to see if all measures are in the same system. No conversion is necessary.

Step 2. Use the formula $\dfrac{D}{OH} \times Q$ and label all parts:

$$\frac{\text{¼ gr}}{\text{½ gr}} \times 1 \text{ ml} = \text{¼} \div \text{½} \times 1$$

Note: To divide fractions, invert the divisor and multiply. Therefore:

$$\text{¼} \div \text{½} = \text{¼} \times \text{²⁄₁} = \text{²⁄₄} = \text{½}$$
$$\text{½} \times 1 = \text{½} = 0.5 \text{ ml}$$

Step 3. Check for reasonableness. A dose of 0.5 ml is within normal limits.

EXAMPLE 5

The order reads atropine sulfate 0.4 mg IM on call to surgery. The ampoule is labeled atropine sulfate 1.0 mg/ml.

Step 1. Check to see if all measures are in the same system. No conversion is necessary.

Step 2. Use the formula $\dfrac{D}{OH} \times Q$ and label all parts:

$$\frac{0.4 \text{ mg}}{1.0 \text{ mg}} \times 1 \text{ ml} = 0.4 \div 1.0 = 1\overline{)0.4}^{\,0.4}$$
$$0.4 \times 1 \text{ ml} = 0.4 \text{ ml}$$

Step 3. Check for reasonableness. A dose of 0.4 ml is within normal limits.

CAUTIONS FOR THE BASIC CALCULATION METHOD

1. *Label* all parts of the formula.
2. Use the *same label* for desired and on-hand doses.
3. Use the *same label* for the quantity and the answer (the amount to be given).
4. *Reduce fractions* to lowest terms before dividing.
5. *Multiply by the quantity* after dividing.
6. Take *extra care* with *decimals*.
7. *Convert* fractions to decimals. *Round off* decimals to one decimal place.
8. *Verify the accuracy* of calculations with an instructor.
9. *Question* the answer if not within normal limits (e.g., less than ½ tab, more than 2 tabs, or more than 2 ml for injection).

Method 2: Ratio and Proportion

A *ratio* describes a relationship between two numbers.

Example: 1 g : 15 gr

A *proportion* consists of two ratios which are equal.

Example: 1 g : 15 gr = 2g : 30 gr

Always label each term in the equation. The terms of each ratio must be in the same sequence. In the examples above, you will see that the first term of each ratio is labeled g and the second term of each ratio is labeled gr.

To solve a problem with the ratio and proportion method, set up the formula with the known terms on the left and the desired and unknown terms on the right. Use X to represent the unknown. Label all terms.

For example, we know that 1,000 mg is equal to 1 g (known). We need to administer 500 mg (desired) and do not know how many grams are equivalent (unknown = X). To convert a dosage from one system to another when a table of metric and apothecary equivalents (such as Table 5.4) is unavailable, set up the problem as a proportion:

$$\underset{\text{of measure}}{Known\ \text{unit}} : \underset{\text{equivalent}}{Known} = \underset{\text{of measure}}{desired\ \text{unit}} : \underset{\text{equivalent}}{unknown}$$

1,000 mg : 1 g = 500 mg : X g

└─── means ───┘
└──────── extremes ────────┘

To solve the problem, multiply the two outer terms, or extremes, and then multiply the two inner terms, or means. Using our example:

$$1,000\ X = 500 = 1,000 \overline{\smash{\big)}\,500.0}^{\,0.5}$$
$$X = 0.5\ \text{g}$$

We now know that our desired dose, 500 mg, is equal to 0.5 g.

When the dose ordered differs from the dose on hand, the problem can be solved simply by completing three basic steps:

1. Verify that all measures are in the same system. Convert if necessary by using a table of metric and apothecary equivalents if available or by using the ratio and proportion method if the equivalent is unknown.
2. Set up the problem as a proportion, label all terms, and complete the calculations:

$$\underset{\text{on hand}}{\text{Dose}} : \underset{\text{quantity}}{\text{known}} = \underset{\text{desired}}{\text{dose}} : \underset{\text{quantity}}{\text{unknown}}$$

Note: The answer should be stated as whole number or a decimal. Convert fractions to decimals and round off to one decimal place.

3. Check the accuracy of your answer for reasonableness and also have someone else verify your calculations.

EXAMPLE 1

The preoperative order reads Demerol 60 mg IM on call. The narcotics locker contains ampoules labeled meperidine (Demerol) 100 mg/2 ml.

Step 1. Verify that all measures are in the same system. No conversion is necessary.

Step 2. Set up the problem as a proportion and label all terms:

$$\begin{array}{ccc} \text{Drug} & \text{known} & \text{dose} & \text{unknown} \\ \text{on hand} & \text{quantity} & \text{desired} & \text{quantity} \end{array}$$

$$100 \text{ mg} : 2 \text{ ml} = 60 \text{ mg} : X \text{ ml}$$

$$100 X = 120 = 100 \overline{)120.0}^{1.2}$$

$$X = 1.2 \text{ ml}$$

Step 3. Check for reasonableness. A dose of 1.2 ml is within normal limits.

EXAMPLE 2

The order reads phenobarbital gr ¾ PO q6h. On-hand phenobarbital tablets are labeled gr 1½/tab.

Step 1. Verify that all measures are in the same system. No conversion is necessary.

Step 2. Set up the problem as a proportion and label all terms:

$$\begin{array}{ccc} \text{Dose} & \text{known} & \text{dose} & \text{unknown} \\ \text{on hand} & \text{quantity} & \text{desired} & \text{quantity} \end{array}$$

$$1\frac{1}{2} \text{ gr} : 1 \text{ tab} = \frac{3}{4} \text{ gr} : X \text{ tabs}$$

$$1\frac{1}{2} X = \frac{3}{4} \text{ or } \frac{3}{4} \div 1\frac{1}{2}$$

Note: When dividing fractions, invert the divisor:

$$\frac{3}{4} \div \frac{3}{2} = \frac{3}{4} \times \frac{2}{3} = \frac{1}{2}$$

$$X = \frac{1}{2} \text{ tab}$$

Step 3. Check for reasonableness. A dose of ½ tab is reasonable. When dividing tablets, cut carefully on scored line with knife or file for exact dosage.

EXAMPLE 3

The medicine drawer contains ampoules labeled atropine sulfate 0.4 mg/ml. The preoperative order reads atropine sulfate gr ⅟₂₀₀ IM on call.

Step 1. Verify that all measures are in the same system. Conversion is necessary. Consult a table of equivalents and/or set up the problem as a proportion:

$$\begin{array}{ccc} \text{Known unit} & \text{known} & \text{desired unit} & \text{unknown} \\ \text{of measure} & \text{equivalent} & \text{of measure} & \text{equivalent} \end{array}$$

$$1 \text{ mg} : \frac{1}{60} \text{ gr} = 0.4 \text{ mg} : X \text{ gr}$$

$$1 X = \frac{1}{60} \times \frac{4}{10}$$

$$X = \frac{1}{150} \text{ gr}$$

Step 2. Set up the problem as a proportion and label all terms:

$$\begin{array}{ccc} \text{Dose} & \text{known} & \text{dose} & \text{unknown} \\ \text{on hand} & : \text{quality} & = \text{desired} & : \text{quantity} \end{array}$$

$$\frac{1}{150} \text{ gr} : 1 \text{ ml} = \frac{1}{200} \text{ gr} : X \text{ ml}$$

$$\frac{1}{150} X = \frac{1}{200} = \frac{1}{200} \div \frac{1}{150}$$

$$X = \frac{3}{4} = 0.75 = 0.8 \text{ ml}$$

Note: Convert fractions to decimals and round off to one decimal place.

Step 3. Check for reasonableness. A dose of 0.8 ml is within normal limits.

EXAMPLE 4
The order reads morphine sulfate gr ⅙ IM q4h PRN for pain. The narcotics locker contains ampoules labeled morphine sulfate 15 mg/ml.

Step 1. Verify that all measures are in the same system. Conversion is necessary. Consult a table of equivalents and/or set up the problem as a proportion. Label all terms:

$$\begin{array}{ccc} \text{Known unit} & \text{known} & \text{desired unit} & \text{unknown} \\ \text{of measure} & : \text{equivalent} & = \text{of measure} & : \text{quantity} \end{array}$$

$$1 \text{ gr} : 60 \text{ mg} = \frac{1}{6} \text{ gr} : X \text{ mg}$$

$$1 X = 60 \times \frac{1}{6}$$

$$X = 10 \text{ mg}$$

Step 2. Set up the problem as a proportion and label all terms:

$$\begin{array}{ccc} \text{Dose} & \text{known} & \text{dose} & \text{unknown} \\ \text{on hand} & : \text{quantity} & = \text{desired} & : \text{quantity} \end{array}$$

$$15 \text{ mg} : 1 \text{ ml} = 10 \text{ mg} : X \text{ ml}$$

$$15 X = 10 = 15 \overline{)10.00} \quad \begin{array}{c} 0.66 = 0.7 \end{array}$$

$$X = 0.7 \text{ ml} \quad \frac{90}{100}$$

Step 3. Check for reasonableness. A dose of 0.7 ml is within normal limits.

EXAMPLE 5
The physician orders Benadryl elixir 25 mg q12h. The bottle in the medicine cupboard is labeled 12.5 mg/d.

Step 1. Verify that all measures are in the same system. No conversion is necessary.

Step 2. Write the problem as a proportion and label each term:

$$\frac{\text{Dose}}{\text{on hand}} : \frac{\text{known}}{\text{quantity}} = \frac{\text{dose}}{\text{desired}} : \frac{\text{unknown}}{\text{quantity}}$$

$$12.5 \text{ mg} : 1 \text{ dr} = 25 \text{ mg} : X \text{ dr}$$

$$12.5 \, X = 25 = 12.5. \, \overline{)25.0.} \,^{2}$$

$$X = 2 \text{ dr}$$

Step 3. Check for reasonableness. The dose 2 dr is within normal limits.

CAUTIONS FOR THE RATIO AND PROPORTION METHOD

1. *Label* all parts of the equation.
2. The ratio on the *left* contains the *known* quantity, and the ratio on the *right* contains the *desired* and *unknown* quantities.
3. Terms of the second ratio must be in the *same sequence* as those in the first ratio.
4. *Multiply* the *extremes first* and then the means.
5. Take *extra care* with *decimals*.
6. *Convert* fractions to decimals. *Round off* decimals to one decimal place.
7. *Label* the answer.
8. *Verify the accuracy* of calculations with an instructor.
9. *Question* any unusual dosage not within normal limits (e.g., less than ½ tab, more than 2 tabs, or more than 2 ml for injection).

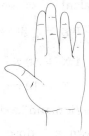

STOP!
Check your knowledge of this chapter before going any further.

CHAPTER REVIEW QUIZ

Show your work. Label and circle your answer:

1. The physician orders procaine penicillin G 500,000 U. Available is Bicillin in a vial labeled penicillin G procaine 300,000 U/ml. How much should you draw into the syringe?

2. The medication order reads Demerol 60 mg IM on call. The narcotic drawer contains vials labeled meperidine (Demerol) 75 mg/ml. How much should you draw into the syringe?

3. Lasix is available in 40-mg tablets. The order reads Lasix 60 mg PO qAM. How many tablets should you give?

4. Atropine 0.6 mg is ordered preoperatively. Available vials of atropine are labeled 0.4 mg/ml. How much should you draw into the syringe?

5. ASA 600 mg q6h is ordered. Aspirin on hand is labeled 5 gr/tab. How many tablets should you give?

6. Morphine sulfate 20 mg PRN q4h is ordered. The narcotic locker contains 2-ml vials labeled morphine sulfate 15 mg/ml. How much should you draw into the syringe?

7. The medication order reads heparin 7,500 U IV stat. Vials available in the medication cupboard labeled heparin 10,000 U/ml. How many milliliters should you draw into the syringe?

8. Digoxin elixir is available in 50 μg/ml. The physician orders 75 μg Lanoxin qd. How many milliliters should you give?

9. The physician orders prednisone 7.5 mg qd. Prednisone is available in 5-mg and 10-mg scored tablets, which can be broken in half. Which strength tablet and how many tablets should you give?

10. Amoxicillin suspension 750 mg q8h is ordered. Liquid medication available is labeled 250 mg/5 ml. How many milliliters should you give?

11. Calcium carbonate 1,000 mg qd is prescribed, to be given in divided doses bid. Available tablets contain calcium 250 mg/tab. How many tablets should be taken each time?

12. Robitussin A-C contains 10 mg of codeine in each teaspoon (5 ml). If 2 tsp Robitussin A-C is prescribed q4h, how much codeine should be contained in each dose?

7

Responsibilities and Principles of Drug Administration

OBJECTIVES

Upon completion of this chapter, the student will be able to:

1. Describe four responsibilities of the health care provider in safe administration of medications.
2. List the five Rights of Medication Administration.
3. Explain moral, ethical, and legal responsibilities regarding medication errors.
4. Cite three instances of medication administration that require documentation.
5. Explain the rights of the health care worker to question or refuse to administer medications.

Responsible Drug Administration

The safe and accurate administration of medications requires knowledge, judgment, and skill. The *responsibilities* of the health care provider in this vital area include:

1. Adequate, up-to-date *information* about all medications to be administered, including purpose, potential side effects, cautions and contraindications, and possible interactions.
2. *Wisdom* and judgment to accurately *assess* the patient's needs for medications, to *evaluate* the response to medications, and to plan appropriate interventions as indicated.
3. *Skill in delivery* of the medication accurately, in the best interests of the patient, and with adequate documentation.
4. *Patient education* to provide the necessary information to the patient and family about why, how, and when medications are to be administered and potential side effects and precautions with administration by the layperson.

Responsibility for safe administration of medications requires that the health care worker be familiar with every medication before administration. Knowledge of the typical and most frequently used drugs of the systems (as described in Part II of this text) is imperative. However, this is only a framework upon which to build and add other knowledge of new drugs or new effects as changes in medicine become known. Unfamiliar drugs should *never* be administered. Resources such as the *PDR,* the *USP/NF,* package inserts, and pharmacists must be consulted *before* administration in order to become familiar with the desired effect, potential side effects, precautions and contraindications, and possible interactions with other drugs or with foods.

Responsibility for safe administration of medicines requires *complete planning* for patient care, including prior *assessment, interventions,* and *evaluations* of the results of drug therapy. Assessment involves taking a complete history, including all medical conditions (e.g., pregnancy or illness), allergies, and all other medications in use, including over-the-counter drugs. Assessment also involves careful observation of the patient's vital signs, posture, skin temperature and color, and facial expression before and after drug administration. Appropriate interventions require judgment in timing, discontinuing medicine if required, and taking steps to counteract adverse reactions, as well as knowing what and when to report to the physician. Evaluation and documentation of results also play a vital role for all health care providers, including the physician, in planning effective drug therapy.

The safe administration of medications necessitates training to develop skills in delivery of medications. The goal is to maximize the effectiveness of the drug with the least discomfort to the patient. Sensitivity to the unique needs of each patient is encouraged (e.g., awareness of difficulty swallowing or impaired movement that could affect administration of medications).

Patient education is an essential part of the safe administration of medicines. If the patient is to benefit from drug therapy, he or she must understand the importance of taking the medicine in the proper dosage, on time, and in the proper way. Information for patients should be in language they understand, with instruction both verbal and written, as well as demonstrations of techniques when indicated.

Administration of medication carries moral, ethical, and legal responsibilities. Some rules and regulations vary with the institution, agency, or office. When in doubt, consult those in authority — supervisors or administrators — administration or procedure books. However, documentation on the patient's record is always required for all medicines given, as well as for patient education provided. In addition, controlled substances given must also be recorded in a narcotics record.

Meticulous care in preparation and administration of medications reduces the chances of error. However, if a mistake is made, it is of the utmost importance to report it immediately to the one in charge so that corrective action can be taken for the patient's welfare. The patient's record should reflect the corrective action taken for justification in case of legal proceedings. An incident report must also be completed as a legal requirement. Failure to report errors appropriately can jeopardize the patient's welfare, as well as increase the possibility of civil suits against the health care provider and/or the risk of loss of professional license or certificate. Honesty is not only the best policy, it is the *only* policy for moral, ethical, and legal reasons.

Principles of Administration

When preparing to administer medications, several basic principles should always be kept in mind:

1. *Cleanliness.* Essential to safe administration of medicines. Always wash hands before handling medicines and be sure preparation area is also clean and neat.
2. *Organization.* Necessary for safe administration of medicines. Always be sure medications and supplies are in the appropriate area and in adequate supply. When stock drugs are used, they should be reordered immediately.
3. *Preparation area.* Should be well-lighted and away from distracting influences.

Guidelines to review before giving medicines are called the five Rights of Medication Administration (Fig. 7.1):

1. Right medication
2. Right amount
3. Right time
4. Right route
5. Right patient

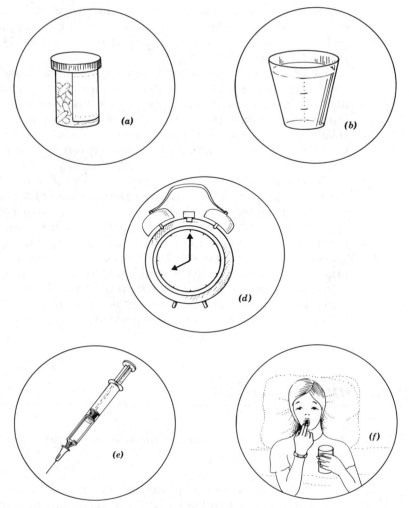

Figure 7.1   *The five Rights of Medication Administration.* (a) *Right medication;* (b) *right amount;* (c) *right time;* (d) *right route;* (e) *right patient.*

RIGHT MEDICATION

You can confirm that you have the right medication by carefully comparing the name of the drug prescribed (on the physician's order sheet, prescription blank, medication record, or medicine card) with the label on the package, bottle, or unit-dose packet (medications with each dose separately sealed in an individual paper, foil, plastic, or glass container). *Never* give medication in which the name of the medicine is obscured in any way. Some drugs have names that sound or look similar (e.g., digoxin and digitoxin, or Inderal and Isuprel), and therefore it is essential to scrutinize every letter in the name when comparing the medicine ordered with the medicine on hand. Accuracy can be facilitated by placing the unit-dose packet next to the name of the drug ordered on the patient's record, while comparing the drug ordered with the drug on hand.

If there is any question about the drug order because of handwriting, misspelling, inappropriateness, allergies, or interactions, you have the *right* and *responsibility to question* the physician and/or the pharmacist.

Never give medications that someone else has prepared. *Never* leave medications at the bedside unless specifically ordered by the doctor (e.g., nitroglycerin tablets and contraceptives are frequently ordered to be left with the patient for self-administration). If the patient is unable to take a medication when you present it, the medication must be returned (in an unopened packet) to the patient's drawer in the medicine cart or medicine room. Never open the unit-dose packet until the patient is prepared to take the medicine.

RIGHT AMOUNT

Administering the right amount of the drug is extremely important. Drug dosage ordered must be compared *very carefully* with the dose listed on the label of the package, bottle, or unit dose packet. Here again, accuracy can be facilitated by placing the unit-dose packet next to the written order on the patient's record while comparing the dose ordered with the dose on hand.

The three different systems of measurement (household, apothecary, and metric) were discussed in Chapter 5. It is important to consult a table of equivalents (Table 5.4), if necessary, to convert from one system to another. Directions for calculation of different drug doses were presented in Chapter 6. Drug calculations are infrequent with unit-dose packaging. However, if it is necessary to compute calculations, such calculations must be checked by another trained health care worker, pharmacist, or doctor to verify accuracy. Be especially careful when the dose is expressed in decimals or fractions. Always recheck the dose if less than one tablet or more than one tablet are requried, or with less than one milliliter or more than one milliliter for injection. An unusual dosage should alert you to the possibility of error. Those who administer medications have the right, as well as the responsibility, to question any dosage that is unusual or seems inappropriate for the individual patient. Remember that drug action is influenced by the condition of the patient, metabolism, age, weight, sex, and psychological state (see Chapter 3). The health care worker has the responsibility of reporting the results of careful assessment and observations in order to assist the physician in prescribing the right dosage for each patient.

Directions for measurement and preparation of the right dose are described in Chapters 8 and 9. An important part of patient education includes complete instructions about the importance of preparing and taking the right amount of medicine prescribed by the physician.

RIGHT TIME

The time for administration of medications is an important part of the drug *dosage*, which includes the amount, frequency, and number of doses of medication to be administered. For maximum effectiveness, drugs must be given on a prescribed schedule. The physician's order specifies the number of times per day the medicine is to be administered (e.g., bid, or twice a day). Some medications need to be maintained at a specific level in the blood and are therefore prescribed at regular intervals around the clock (e.g., q4h, or every 4 hours). Some medications, such as antibiotics, are more effective on an empty stomach and are therefore prescribed ac (before meals). Medications that are irritating to the stomach are be ordered pc (after meals). Drugs that cause sedation are more frequently prescribed at hs (hour of sleep). If the physician does not prescribe a specific time for administration of a drug, the health care worker arranges an appropriate schedule, taking into consideration the purpose, action, and side effects of the medication. Patient education includes instruction about the right time to take specific medicines and why.

RIGHT ROUTE

The route of administration is important because of its effect on degree of absorption, speed of drug action, and side effects. Many drugs can be administered in a variety of ways (see Chapter 4). The physician's order specifies the route of administration. If no route is specified, the oral route is used unless conditions warrant otherwise (e.g., nausea, vomiting, or difficulty swallowing). Those administering medications have the right and responsibility to question the appropriateness of a route based on assessment and observation of the patient. Change of route may be indicated because of the patient's condition. However, the route of administration may not be changed without the physician's order.

RIGHT PATIENT

The patient who is to receive the medication must be identified by use of certain techniques to reduce the chance of error. The patient's wrist identification band should be checked *first*, and then the patient should be called by name, *before* administering the medication. If the patient questions the medication or the dosage, recheck the order and the medicine before giving it.

THE "SIXTH RIGHT"

After completing the steps outlined in the five Rights of Administration, there is one further important step required. Sometimes called the "Sixth Right," another essential duty is *documentation*. Every medication given must be recorded on the patient's record, along with *dose, time, route,* and *location* of injections. If the medication is given on a PRN (as necessary) basis (e.g., for pain), notation should also be made on the patient's record of the effectiveness of the medication. The person administering the medication must also sign or initial the record after administration (the policy of each facility determines the exact procedure to be followed). The accuracy of medication documentation is a very important legal responsibility. At times, patients' records are examined in court, and the accuracy of medication documentation can be a critical factor in some legal judgments.

Documentation also includes the recording of narcotics administered on the special controlled substances record kept with the narcotics. If narcotics are destroyed because of partial dosage, cancellation, or error, two health care workers must sign as witnesses of the disposal of the drug (the policy about documentation of narcotics may vary with the agency).

In summary, safe and effective administration of medications involves current drug information; technical and evaluation skills; and moral, ethical, and legal responsibilities. Guidelines include the five Rights of Medication Administration. The right documentation is also an essential responsibility. In addition, the health care worker has the right and responsibility to question any medication order that is confusing or illegible or that seems inappropriate, and the right to refuse to administer any medication that is not in the best interests of the patient. The primary concern in administration of medications is the welfare of the patient.

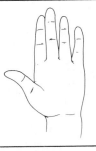

STOP!
Check your knowledge of this chapter before going any further.

CHAPTER REVIEW QUIZ

Complete the statements by filling in the blanks:

1. Before administering any medication, you should have the following information about the drug:

   _____   _____

   _____   _____

2. Before administering any medication, you should have the following three pieces of information about the patient:

   _____   _____

   other _____

3. Assessment of the patient's need for pain medication and reactions to drugs includes observation of the following four signs:

   _____   _____

   _____   _____

4. Patient education about medication should include the following four pieces of information:

   _____   _____

   _____   _____

5. When administering a controlled substance, documentation is necessary in two places:

   _____

   _____

6. Documentation of an injection given for pain should include the following five pieces of information:

   _____   _____

   _____   _____

   _____

7. Name the five Rights of Drug Administration:

   _____

   _____

   _____

   _____

   _____

8. Medication errors must be reported immediately, and documentation includes recording the information in the following two areas:

_____

_____

8

Administration by the Gastrointestinal Route

OBJECTIVES

Upon completion of this chapter, the student will be able to:

1. Describe the advantages and disadvantages of administering medications orally, by nasogastric tube, and rectally.
2. Explain appropriate action when patient is NPO, refuses medication, vomits medication, or has allergies.
3. List special precautions in preparation of timed-release spansules, enteric-coated tablets, and oral suspensions.
4. Demonstrate measurement of liquid medications with medicine cup and syringe.
5. Demonstrate proficiency in administering medications orally, by nasogastric tube, and rectally.
6. Satisfactorily complete all of the activities listed on the checklists.

Medications are administered by the gastrointestinal route more often than any other way. Gastrointestinal administration includes three categories: oral, nasogastric tube, and rectal.

Advantages of the oral route include:

- Convenience and patient comfort
- Safety, since medication can be retrieved in case of error or intentional overdose
- Economy, since there are few equipment costs

Disadvantages of the oral route include

- Slower onset of absorption and action
- Rate and degree of absorption that vary with gastrointestinal contents and motility
- Some drugs (e.g., insulin and heparin) destroyed by digestive fluids and must be administered by injection
- Cannot be used with nausea or vomiting
- Dangerous to use if patient has difficulty swallowing (dysphagia), because of possible aspiration
- Cannot be used for unconscious patients
- Cannot be used if patient is NPO (e.g., before surgery or while fasting for a laboratory test or X-ray examination)

Administration of medications by nasogastric tube is sometimes ordered when the patient is unable to swallow for prolonged periods of time because of illness, trauma, surgery, or unconsciousness. Medications are usually administered intravenously when these conditions exist for short periods of time. *Advantages of the nasogastric tube* include:

- Ability to bypass the mouth and pharynx when necessary
- Elimination of numerous injections

The *disadvantage of the nasogastric tube* with a conscious patient is the discomfort of the tube in the nose and throat for prolonged periods of time.

Medications are sometimes administered by the rectal route when nausea or vomiting is present, or the patient is unconscious or unable to swallow. *Advantages of the rectal route* include:

- Bypassing the action of digestive enzymes
- Avoidance of irritation to the upper GI tract

Disadvantages of the rectal route include:

- Many medications are unavailable in suppository form.
- Some patients have difficulty retaining suppositories (e.g., the elderly and children).
- Prolonged use of some rectal suppositories can cause rectal irritation (e.g., aminophyllin).
- Absorption may be irregular or incomplete if feces are present.

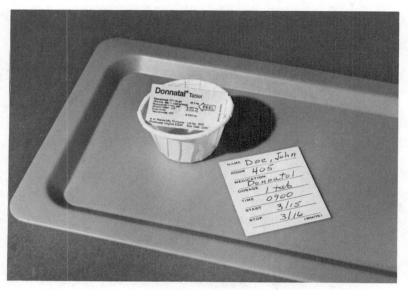

Figure 8.1 *Medicine in a cup is placed on a tray with patient identification.*

Administration of Medications Orally

GUIDELINES FOR ADMINISTRATION OF ORAL MEDICATIONS

1. Wash your hands.
2. Locate appropriate medication sheet and check for completeness of the order (i.e., date, patient's name, medication name, dosage, route, and time).
3. Check for special circumstances (e.g., allergies or NPO).
4. Be sure that you know the purpose of the drug, possible side effects, contraindications, cautions, interactions, and normal dosage range. If unfamiliar with the drug, consult a reference book for this information.
5. Select appropriate receptacle in which to place medication (i.e., paper medicine cup for tablets or capsules and plastic medicine cup for liquids). Place medicine cup and patient identification card on tray (Fig. 8.1).
6. Locate medication in medication cupboard or medication cart drawer and compare the label against the medication sheet for the five Rights of Medication Administration: right medicine, right amount, right time, right route, and right patient (Fig. 8.2).
7. If the dose ordered differs from the dose on hand, complete calculations on paper and check for accuracy with instructor.
8. Prepare the dosage as ordered. Do not open unit dose packages until you are with the patient (Fig. 8.3). If medication is liquid, see "Preparation of Liquid Medication" later in this section.
9. Take tray to patient and place it on table nearby.
10. Check patient's identification bracelet (Fig. 8.4).

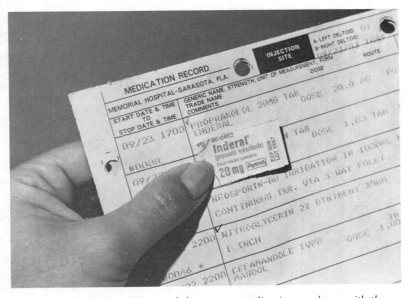

Figure 8.2   *Compare name and dosage on medication package with the medication sheet.*

11. Call patient by name and explain what you are doing. Answer any questions. Recheck medication order if patient expresses any doubts. Use this opportunity for patient education about the medication.
12. Monitor patient's vital signs if required for specific medication (e.g., apical pulse or respiration).
13. Open unit-dose package and place container in the patient's hand. Avoid touching the medication (Fig. 8.5).
14. Provide full glass of water and assist the patient as necessary (e.g., raise the head of the bed and providing drinking straw if required).

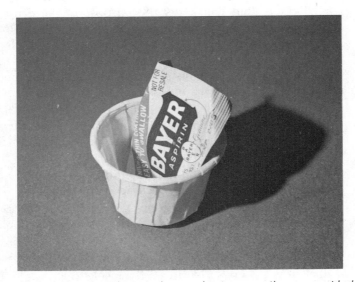

Figure 8.3   *Keep the unit dose packet intact until you are with the patient.*

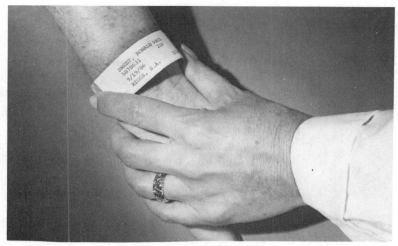

Figure 8.4 *Check identification to be sure it is the right patient.*

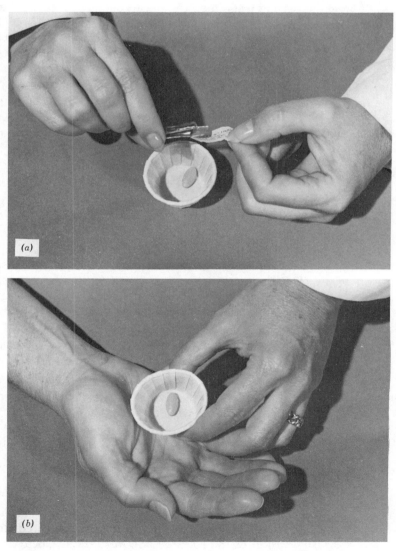

Figure 8.5 *Do not touch medicine. (a) Open the unit dose packet and drop the tablet in a cup. (b) Place the cup containing the medicine in the patient's hand.*

15. Stay with the patient until the medication has been swallowed. Make the patient comfortable before you leave the room.

16. Discard used medicine cup and wrappers in wastebasket.

17. Return clean tray to medicine cart or medicine room.

18. Record the medication, dosage, time, and your signature or initials in the correct place on patient's record.

19. Document on patient's record and report if a medication is withheld or refused and the reason. Record and report any unusual circumstances associated with administration or any adverse side effects.

SPECIAL CONSIDERATIONS FOR ORAL ADMINISTRATION

1. If patient is NPO, check with the person in charge regarding appropriate procedure, based on reason for NPO. If patient is fasting for laboratory X-ray tests, medication can usually be given at a later time with possible modification of time schedule. If patient is NPO for surgery, nausea, or dysphagia, the doctor may need to be consulted regarding a change of route. *Do not* omit the medications completely without specific instructions to that effect. Abrupt withdrawal of some medications, for example, phenytoin (Dilantin) or diazepam (Valium), may lead to seizures.

2. Always check the patient's record for *allergies* and be aware of the components of combination products. Patients with a history of allergy should be watched carefully for possible drug reactions when any new medication is administered.

3. Give the most important medicine first.

4. Elevate the patient's head, if not contraindicated by the patient's condition, to aid in swallowing.

5. Stay with the patient until the medication is swallowed. *Do not* leave the medication at bedside or in the patient's possession unless ordered by physician.

6. Administer oral medications with water, unless ordered otherwise. *Do not* give medicine with fruit juice, milk, or any other liquid unless indicated by specific directions. The absorption of many medicines (e.g., antibiotics) is inhibited by interaction with acid or alkaline products.

7. Medications whose action depends on contact with the mucous membranes of the mouth or throat (e.g., topical anesthetics or fungicides) should *not* be administered with any fluid or food.

8. *Do not* open or crush timed-release capsules or enteric-coated tablets.

9. If tablets must be divided, place on paper towel and cut with the knife on score marks only, for accuracy. *Do not* break by hand.

10. When removing tablets or capsules from a stock bottle, pour into lid and from there into medicine cup. *Do not* touch tablets or capsules.

11. *Do not* administer any medication that is discolored, has precipitated, is contaminated, or is outdated.

12. If a patient is NPO, refuses the medication, or vomits within 20–30 min. of taking the medication, always report this to the person in charge. A written order from the physician is required to change either the medication or the route of administration. Document on the patient's record the time of emesis and appearance of the emesis.

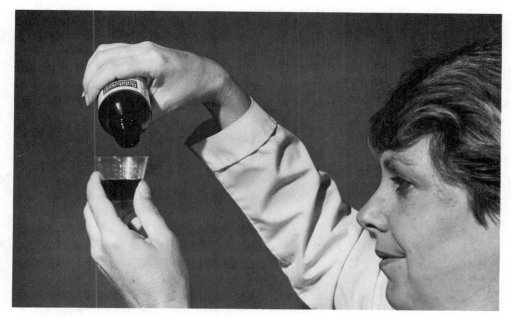

Figure 8.6 *Hold the medicine bottle with label side up and medicine cup at eye level, with thumbnail marking measurement.*

13. If the patient refuses a medication, determine the reason. Report the refusal and reason to the person in charge and record all information on patient's record.

14. Tablets (unless enteric-coated) may be crushed with mortar and pestle. Capsules (except timed-release capsules) may be opened and the contents mixed with applesauce or ice cream to facilitate administration for patients with difficulty swallowing (e.g., children and the elderly). Check diet to be sure these foods are allowed.

PREPARATION OF LIQUID MEDICATIONS

Follow the "Guidelines for Administration of Oral Medications," at the beginning of this section. Preparation of *liquid medications* requires these additional steps:

1. Shake bottle if indicated. Remove cap and place cap upside down on table.
2. Hold medicine bottle with label side upward to prevent smearing of label while pouring (Fig. 8.6).
3. In other hand, hold medicine cup at eye level and place thumbnail on level to which medication will be poured (Fig. 8.6).
4. While holding the medicine cup straight at eye level, pour the prescribed amount of medication.
5. Replace cap on bottle.
6. Compare the information on the medication sheet against the label on the stock bottle and the quantity of drug in the cup.
7. Replace medication bottle in cupboard or medicine cart.

8. Recheck the five Rights of Medication Administration.
9. Proceed with the "Guidelines for Administration of Oral Medications."

When administering liquid medication to someone who is unable to drink from a cup (e.g., infants and persons with wired jaws), a syringe may be used. Follow the "Guidelines for Administration of Oral Medications." Administration of *liquid medications orally via syringe* requires these additional steps:

1. Pour prescribed medication into medicine cup.
2. Withdraw prescribed amount with syringe.
3. Check medication and order using the five Rights of Medication Administration.
4. Identify the patient and elevate the patient's head.
5. Be sure the patient is alert and able to swallow.
6. Place the syringe tip in the pocket between the cheek and the gums. (When administering large amounts of liquid via syringe, it helps to fit a 2-inch length of latex tubing on the syringe tip to facilitate instillation of the medication into the cheek pocket.)
7. Instill the medication slowly to lessen chances of aspiration.
8. Be sure all medication is swallowed before leaving the patient.
9. Proceed with "Guidelines for the Administration of Oral Medications."

Administration of Medications by Nasogastric Tube

A nasogastric tube is not inserted solely for the purpose of administering medication. However, medications are sometimes ordered by this route when a nasogastric tube is in place for tube feeding or for suction. When medications are ordered by nasogastric tube, follow the "Guidelines for Administration of Oral Medications" and "Preparation of Liquid Medications."

Administration of medication by nasogastric tube requires these additional steps:

1. Check the medication order using the five Rights of Medication Administration.
2. Wash hands.
3. Prepare the medication as ordered and take to the patient's room. Be sure the medication is at room temperature.
4. Check identification bracelet, call the patient by name, and explain the procedure. Elevate head of bed, if not contraindicated.
5. Hold the end of the tube up and remove the clamp, plug, or adapter.
6. Make sure that the tube is properly placed in the stomach by using at least two tests (Fig. 8.7):
   a. Aspirate with bulb or piston syringe for stomach contents to verify correct placement. Then flush tube with normal saline solution.
   b. Place a stethoscope over the patient's stomach, attach the syringe to the tube, and inject about 15 cc of air. If you hear a swooshing sound, air has entered the stomach, verifying correct placement.

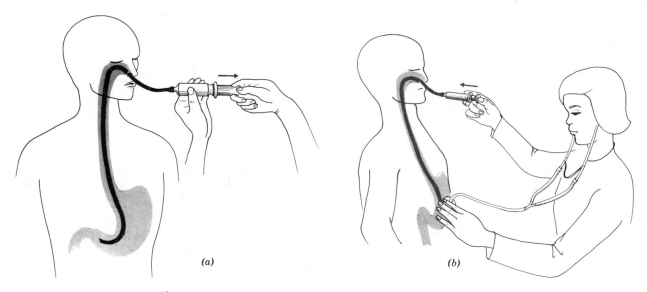

Figure 8.7 *Test for correct placement of nasogastric tube. (a) Aspirate with syringe. (b) Listen with stethoscope as you inject 15 cc of air.*

7. Clamp the tube with your fingers by bending it over upon itself or by pinching it. While tube is closed, remove plunger or bulb from syringe, leaving syringe attached firmly to tubing (Fig. 8.8*a*).

8. Pour medication into syringe. Release or unclamp the tubing and let medication flow through by gravity. Never force fluids down a nasogastric tube (Fig. 8.8*b*). Watch the patient during the procedure and stop immediately at any sign of discomfort by pinching the tube. Holding the syringe too high causes fluid to run in too quickly, possibly causing nausea and vomiting.

9. Before the syringe empties completely, flush the tube by adding 30–50 ml of water to the syringe (Fig. 8.8*c*). If the patient's input and output are being monitored, be sure to add this amount to the patient's record.

10. After the water has run in, pinch the tube, remove the syringe, and clamp or plug the tube. If the patient is on suction, be sure to leave suction turned *off* for at least 30 min until medication is absorbed.

11. Position patient on right side and/or elevate head of bed to encourage the stomach to empty. Make the patient comfortable.

12. Proceed with "Guidelines for the Administration of Oral Medications" for documentation.

Administration of Medications Rectally

Medications are sometimes ordered to be administered by the rectal route. The medicine may be in suppository form or in liquid form to be administered as a retention enema. This treatment is more effective with the patient's cooperation. Tact and consideration are required for successful administration of rectal med-

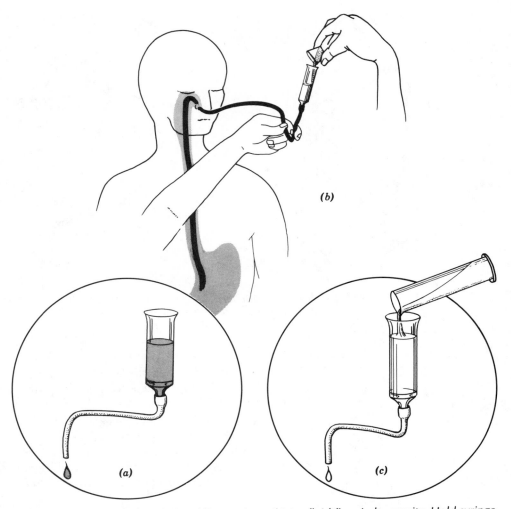

Figure 8.8 (a) *Close tube before filling syringe.* (b) *Let fluid flow in by gravity. Hold syringe at level of patient's shoulder.* (c) *Flush tube with water.*

ications. Remember to respect the patient's dignity and privacy by closing the door and curtains completely. Do not expose the patient unnecessarily.

The retention enema is administered in the same way as a cleansing enema. However, the retention enema must be retained approximately 30 min or more for absorption of the medication. Therefore, the patient is instructed to lie quietly on either side to aid in retention. If the patient is uncooperative, unconscious, or has poor sphincter control, the buttocks can be taped together with 2-inch paper adhesive for 30 min. Do not use this method unless absolutely necessary. Remember to treat the patient with dignity. Always explain everything you are doing and why. Even if patients are unconscious or unable to speak, they may be able to hear and cooperate in some way if they understand.

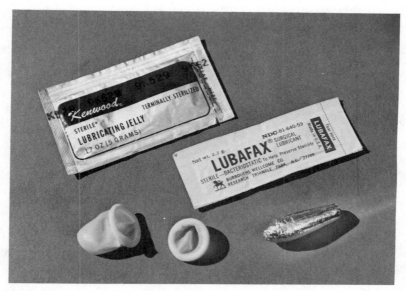

Figure 8.9 *Supplies for administration of a rectal suppository. A finger cot and a small packet of lubricant are required.*

ADMINISTRATION OF RECTAL SUPPOSITORY

1. Wash hands.
2. Check the medication order using the five Rights of Medication Administration.
3. Identify medication (purpose, side effects, contraindications, cautions, and normal dose range). Research information if necessary.
4. Assemble supplies (finger cot or disposable glove and water-soluble lubricant (Fig. 8.9).
5. Select the medication as ordered, checking medication name and dosage again. Some suppositories are stored in a refrigerator, and some may be stored at room temperature, according to manufacturer's instructions.
6. Check patient's identification bracelet, call the patient by name, and explain the procedure. Answer any questions.
7. Close door and curtain completely.
8. Lower the head of the bed if necessary and position the patient on side with upper knee bent. Keep patient covered, exposing only the rectal area (Fig. 8.10).
9. Put on disposable glove, or finger cot on index finger. With infants, use little finger.
10. Remove suppository from wrapper and lubricate the tapered end with water-soluble lubricant.
11. With ungloved hand, separate the patient's buttock's gently so you can see anus.
12. Ask patient to take a deep breath. Insert the lubricated suppository gently into the rectum and push gently with gloved index finger until the suppository has passed the internal sphincter (Fig. 8.11).

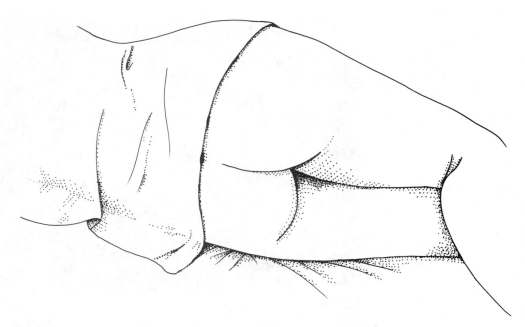

Figure 8.10 *Drape and position patient on side with upper knee bent.*

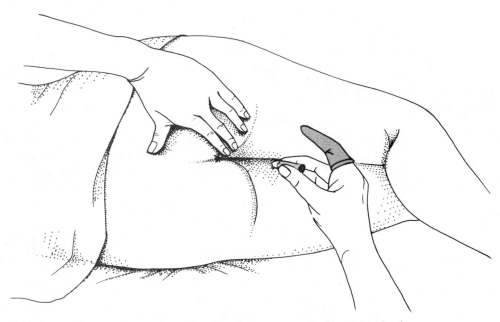

Figure 8.11 *Lubricate tip of suppository and insert it with covered index finger.*

13. Urge the patient to retain the suppository for at least 20 min. If patient is unable to cooperate, hold the buttocks together as required.

14. Remove and dispose of glove or finger cot, turning it inside out as you remove it.

15. Be sure the patient is comfortable, with covers and bed adjusted appropriately.

16. Wash hands.

17. Record the medication in the appropriate place.

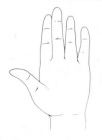

STOP!

Check your knowledge of this chapter before going any further.

CHECKLIST FOR ADMINISTRATION OF ORAL MEDICATIONS

ACTIVITY	RATING	
	S	U
1. Washed hands.		
2. Checked medication sheet for date, dosage, time, route, and allergies.		
3. Identified medication: purpose, side effects, contraindications, cautions, interaction, and normal dosage range.		
4. Selected appropriate medicine cup and placed on tray with patient identification card.		
5. Selected correct medication and checked label against medication sheet for five Rights of Medication Administration.		
6. Calculated correct dosage on paper if necessary.		
7. Placed medication as ordered in cup without opening packet or touching medication. Prepared liquid medication by shaking if necessary, pouring away from label and measuring at eye level.		
8. Identified patient by checking bracelet and calling the patient by name.		
9. Explained procedure to patient and answered any questions about medication.		
10. Checked patient's vital signs if necessary for specific medicine.		
11. Opened unit dose packages and offered medication in container to patient.		
12. Provided drinking water and assisted patient as necessary.		
13. Made patient comfortable and left unit in order.		
14. Recorded medication, dosage, time, and signature or initials on patient's record.		

Note: S, satisfactory; U, unsatisfactory.

CHECKLIST FOR ADMINISTRATION OF RECTAL SUPPOSITORY

ACTIVITY	RATING	
	S	U
1. Washed hands.		
2. Checked the medication order for date, dosage, time, route, and allergies.		
3. Identified medication: purpose, side effects, contraindications, cautions, and normal dosage range.		
4. Assembled supplies: finger cot or glove and lubricant.		
5. Selected correct medication and checked label with medication order for five Rights of Medication Administration.		
6. Identified patient by checking bracelet and calling patient by name.		
7. Explained procedure to patient and answered any questions about medication.		
8. Closed door and curtain.		
9. Positioned patient on side with upper knee bent and only rectal area exposed.		
10. Put on disposable glove, or finger cot on index finger.		
11. Removed wrapping from suppository and lubricated tapered end.		
12. With ungloved hand separated buttocks gently.		
13. Instructed patient to take a deep breath and inserted suppository gently, pushing it past the sphincter.		
14. Instructed patient about retaining the suppository.		
15. Removed glove or finger cot correctly and disposed of them appropriately.		
16. Made patient comfortable and left unit in order.		
17. Washed hands.		
18. Recorded medication, dosage, time, and signature or initials on patient's record.		

Note: S, satisfactory; U, unsatisfactory.

CHAPTER REVIEW QUIZ

1. Name six disadvantages of oral administration compared with administration by injection.

   _____

   _____

   _____

   _____

   _____

   _____

Match the column on left with the appropriate action on the right. Actions may be used more than once:

2. _____ To facilitate swallowing   a. Watch closely for drug reactions

3. _____ If NPO for lab tests   b. Crush tablet, mix with ice cream

4. _____ Patient vomits 15 min after   c. Administer first
         medication

5. _____ Most medications   d. Cannot be opened

6. _____ Patient is allergic to   e. Elevate patient's head
         penicillin

7. _____ Most important medicine   f. Notify person in charge

8. _____ Tablet cannot be   g. Modify schedule, give medicine
         swallowed   later

9. _____ Timed-release capsules   h. Administer with water

10. _____ Dilantin ordered PO,   i. Leave medication at bedside
          patient NPO for surgery

Complete the following statements by filling in the blanks:

When pouring liquid medicine:

11. The bottle should be held _____

12. The medicine cup should be held _____

13. The bottle cap should be placed _____

14. If medication is in suspension, the bottle should first be

_____

When administering medication by nasogastric tube:

15. Check tube placement first with two tests:

_____

_____

Check the appropriate answer:

16. _____ a. Medication should be pushed through the nasogastric tube by pressure on barrel of syringe.
_____ b. Medication should flow through the nasogastric tube by gravity.

17. _____ a. Medication should be cold.
_____ b. Medication should be at room temperature.

18. _____ a. Patient's head should be elevated.
_____ b. Patient should be placed in Trendelenberg position.

19. Name four steps in administration of a rectal suppository that are different from PO administration.

_____

_____

_____

_____

20. Medication documentation should include:

_____

_____

_____

_____

9

Administration by the Parenteral Route

OBJECTIVES

Upon completion of this chapter, the student will be able to:

1. Define parenteral, systemic, local, topical, and transcutaneous delivery systems, and IPPB therapy.
2. Name four parenteral routes with systemic effects.
3. Explain administration via the sublingual and buccal routes, including instructions to the patient.
4. Demonstrate application of nitroglycerin ointment and the transdermal patch.
5. Identify two conditions treated with transcutaneous delivery systems.
6. Compare and contrast advantages and disadvantages of inhalation therapy.
7. Describe patient education for those receiving inhalation therapy with hand-held nebulizers.
8. List cautions when administering IPPB therapy.
9. Identify the three parts of the syringe and the three parts of the needle.
10. Select appropriate-length and correct-gauge needles for various types of injections.
11. List three types of syringes and a purpose for each.
12. Demonstrate drawing up medications from a vial and an ampule.
13. Describe and demonstrate an intradermal injection.
14. Describe and demonstrate a subcutaneous injection.
15. Describe five sites for intramuscular injection.
17. Give purpose and demonstration of Z-track injection.
18. List four types of administration for local effects.

Parenteral routes include any route other than the gastrointestinal tract. The most common form of parenteral administration is injection. However, other routes must be considered as well: the skin, mucous membranes, eyes, ears, and respiratory tract.

Parenteral administration can be understood more easily if the purpose of administration or the effects desired are considered as two categories: systemic and local.

Systemic effects are those affecting the body as a whole, the entire system. The goal of administering drugs for systemic effects is to distribute the medication through the circulatory system to the area requiring treatment. Parenteral routes with systemic effects include (1) sublingual or buccal, (2) transcutaneous (transdermal), (3) inhalations, and (4) injections.

Local effects are those limited to one particular part (location) of the body, with very little, if any, effect on the rest of the body. Medications in this category include:

1. Medications applied to the skin for skin conditions, sometimes called *topical* medications
2. Drugs applied to the mucous membranes to treat that specific tissue
3. Medication instilled in the eyes
4. Medication instilled in the ears

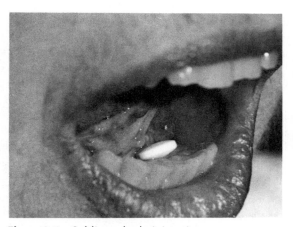

Figure 9.1   *Sublingual administration.*

Sublingual and Buccal Administration

With sublingual administration, the medication is placed under the tongue (Fig. 9.1). The drug is absorbed directly into the circulation through the numerous blood vessels located in the mucosa of this area. With buccal administration, the medication is placed in the pouch between the cheek and the gum at the back of the mouth. The sublingual route is used more commonly than the buccal. Medications absorbed in this way are unaffected by the stomach, intestines, or

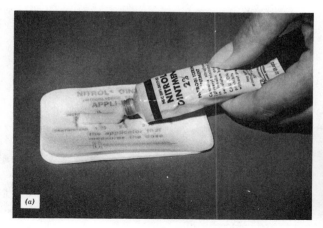 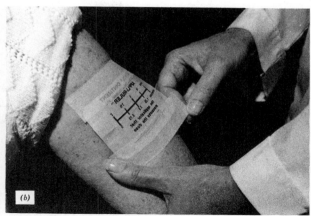

Figure 9.2   *Transdermal administration of nitroglycerin ointment. (a) Ointment is measured on Appli-Ruler paper. (b) Paper containing ointment is applied to the skin.*

liver. Absorption via this route is quite rapid, and therefore this method is used frequently when quick response is required (e.g., with nitroglycerin to treat acute angina pectoris). The constricted coronary blood vessels are usually dilated within a few minutes, bringing quick relief from pain.

PATIENT EDUCATION

For the sublingual or buccal route, include the following instructions:

1. Hold the tablet in place with mouth closed until medication is absorbed.
2. Do not swallow the medication.
3. Do not drink or take food until medication is completely absorbed.

Transcutaneous Drug Delivery System

Transcutaneous, or transdermal, systems deliver the medication to the body by absorption through the skin. Nitroglycerin ointment, for example, is applied to the skin in prescribed amounts every few hours for prevention of angina pectoris. The absorption is slower, and therefore this method is not effective in the treatment of acute angina attacks. Other transcutaneous delivery systems utilize a patch impregnated with a particular medication, applied to the skin, and left in place for continuous absorption. Examples of transcutaneous drug delivery systems include nitroglycerin (Transderm-Nitro), in which the patch is usually left in place for 24 hours in prophylactic treatment of chronic angina; and scopolamine, (Transderm-Scop), in which the patch is placed behind the ear and left in place up to 72 h, as necessary, to prevent motion sickness. Absorption by this method is slower, but the action is more prolonged than with other methods of administration.

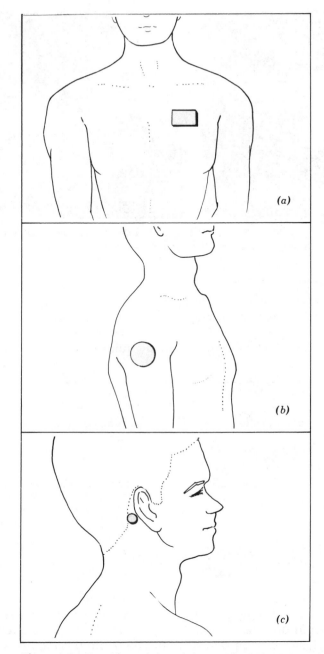

Figure 9.3 *Transdermal drug delivery. Dermal patches vary in size and shape. (a, b) For prevention of angina pectoris; (c) for prevention of motion sickness.*

PATIENT EDUCATION

For those applying transcutaneous systems of administration, include the following instructions. With nitroglycerin ointment (Fig. 9.2):

1. Squeeze the prescribed amount of ointment onto Appliruler paper. When the ointment reaches the correct marking, give the tube a slight twist to cut off the ointment and recap the tube.
2. *Do not* touch the ointment! Absorption of ointment through the skin of the fingers can cause a severe headache.
3. Carefully fold the Appliruler paper lengthwise with the ointment inside.
4. Flatten the folded paper carefully to spread the ointment inside. *Do not* allow the ointment to reach the edges of the paper. Keep paper folded.
5. Rotate sites for application. Appropriate areas include chest, back, upper arms, and upper legs. *Do not* shave the area. Be sure the area is clean, dry, and free of irritation, rash, and abrasion.
6. After the area for application is exposed, open the paper carefully and apply paper to the skin, ointment side down. *Do not* touch ointment. Fasten paper in place with paper tape.
7. Remove previous paper carefully, without touching the inside, and discard in trash container. Cleanse area and inspect skin for any sign of irritation. Report and record any skin changes.
8. Wash hands immediately.

With transdermal sealed drug delivery systems (Fig. 9.3):

1. Select site for administration, rotating areas. Be sure the skin is clean, dry, and free of irritation.
2. Open the packet carefully, pulling the two sides apart *without touching the inside.*
3. Apply the side containing the medication to the skin. Press the adhesive edges down firmly all around. If for any reason the adhesive edges do not stick, fasten in place with paper tape. This is usually unnecessary.
4. Remove previous patch carefully, without touching the inside, and discard in trash container. Cleanse area and inspect skin for irritation.
5. Wash hands immediately.

Inhalation Therapy

Medications are frequently administered by inhalation method, especially to those with chronic pulmonary conditions, such as asthma. Patients may self-administer the medication with a hand-held nebulizer, or the physician may prescribe intermittent positive pressure breathing (IPPB) therapy, to be administered by trained personnel.

Advantages of inhalation therapy include:

1. Rapid action of the drug, with local effects within the respiratory tract.
2. Potent drugs may be given in small amounts, minimizing side effects.
3. Convenience and comfort of the patient.

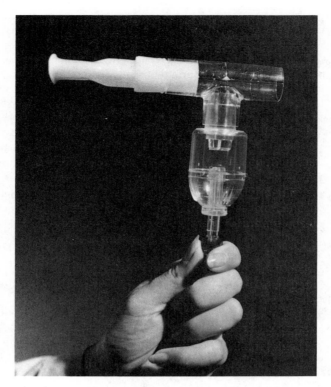

Figure 9.4 *Hand-held nebulizers for administration of medicine by inhalation.*

Disadvantages of inhalation therapy include:

1. Requires cooperation of the patient in proper breathing techniques for effectiveness.
2. Adverse systemic side effects may result rapidly because of extensive absorption capacity of the lungs.
3. Improperly administered, or too frequently administered, inhalations can lead to irritation of the trachea or bronchi, or bronchospasm.
4. Asthmatic patients sometimes become dependent on a nebulizer.
5. If not cleaned properly, the hand-held nebulizer can be a source of infection.

HAND-HELD NEBULIZERS

Patient education is a very important part of inhalation therapy. There are several different varities of hand-held nebulizers on the market (Fig. 9.4), such as the Whirlybird Spinhaler and the metered-dose nebulizer. Instructions for correct use of these devices vary with the particular product. One may specify a quick inhalation; another may require inhaling slowly. Directions may specify tilting the head backward or holding it upright. Each nebulizer comes from the pharmacist with detailed instructions. It is the health care worker's responsibility to be sure that the patient understands and follows the directions correctly for effective therapy.

PATIENT EDUCATION

With use of a nebulizer, include the following instructions:

1. Name of the medication, dosage, and how often it is to be administered.
2. Desired effects and possible adverse side effects (e.g., palpitations, tremor, nervousness, dizziness, headache, nausea, dry mouth, irritated throat, hoarseness, or coughing).
3. Notify the physician if any adverse side effects occur or if the medication seems ineffective. The doctor may want to change the dosage or the medication.
4. Caution *not* to take any other medication, including over-the-counter drugs, without doctor's permission. Many drugs and alcohol can interact with these drugs causing serious side effects.
5. Rising slowly from a reclining position will help prevent dizziness.
6. Rinsing the mouth after inhalation will counteract dry mouth or unpleasant taste.
7. Step-by-step demonstration with the patient, answering all questions.
8. Rinsing equipment after use and storage of medication as indicated on the package.
9. Importance of not smoking.

IPPB THERAPY

Intermittent positive pressure breathing therapy may be ordered by the physician. Health care personnel, such as respiratory therapists or nurses, are specially trained in the use of this equipment (Fig. 9.5).

Cautions with IPPB therapy include:

1. Monitor vital signs closely, watching for a sudden drop in blood pressure, tachycardia, and decreased or shallow respirations.
2. Observe for nausea or distended abdomen.
3. Watch for tremors or dizziness.
4. Assure the patient that coughing after the treatment is to be expected. The goal of the treatment is to aid in coughing up the loosened secretions.
5. Record effectiveness of therapy and any side effects observed or reported by the patient.

Injections

To administer injections, you must be familiar with equipment.

SYRINGES

The syringe has three parts (Fig. 9.6):

1. *Barrel*. The outer, hollow cylinder that holds the medication. It contains the calibrations for measuring the quantity of the medication.

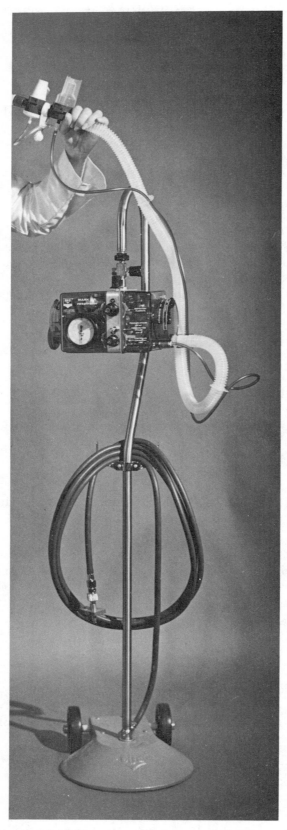

Figure 9.5 Intermittent positive pressure breathing apparatus to deliver medication for inhalation.

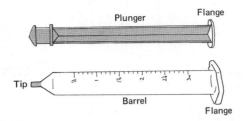

Figure 9.6 *Syringe showing the barrel, the plunger, and the tip.*

2. *Plunger.* The inner, solid rod that fits snugly into the cylinder. Pulling back on the plunger allows solution to be drawn into the syringe. Pushing forward on the plunger ejects solution or air from the syringe.
3. *Tip.* The portion that holds the needle. Most tips are plain. Some larger syringes contain a metal attachment at the tip, called a Luer-lok, which locks the needle in place.

Most syringes are plastic and disposable after one use. Some syringes for special procedures are glass and must be resterilized after use.

NEEDLES

The needle has three parts (Fig. 9.7):

1. *Hub.* The flared end that fits on the tip of the syringe.
2. *Shaft.* The long, hollow tube embedded in the hub. Needles have shafts with different lengths. Shorter needles (½, ⅜, and ⅝ inches) are used for intradermal (into the skin) or subcutaneous (into the tissue just below the skin) injections. Longer needles (1½ and 2 inches) are used for intramuscular (into the muscle) injections. The length of the needle depends on the type of injection and the size of the patient (i.e., shorter needles for children and thin adults and longer needles for larger adults). The gauge is the size of the lumen, or hole, through the needle, or the diameter of the shaft. The gauge is numbered in reverse order (i.e., the thinner needle with the smaller diameter has the larger number, e.g., 25 gauge for subcutaneous injections and 19–21 gauge, a thicker needle with a larger opening for IM or IV injections; see Fig. 9.7). The size of the gauge is determined by the site of the injection and the viscosity of the solution (e.g., blood and oil require a thicker-gauge needle, e.g., 15–18).
3. The tip is the pointed end with a beveled edge.

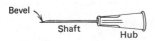

Figure 9.7 *Needle showing the hub, the shaft, and the tip (bevel).*

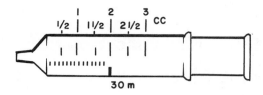

Figure 9.8 *Standard 3-ml syringe.*

Three main types of syringes are used for injections. The type used is determined by the medication and the dosage. The three types are:

1. *Standard syringe.* Used most frequently for subcutaneous or intramuscular injections, calibrated or marked in cubic centimeters (cc) or milliliters (ml) and minims (m) (Fig. 9.8). The most commonly used size is 3 cc or 2½ cc. Larger sizes of 5–50 cc are available for other purposes (e.g., irrigations, withdrawing fluids from the body, and intravenous injections).
2. *Tuberculin (TB) syringe.* Used for intradermal injections of very small amounts of a substance (e.g., testing for tuberculosis or for allergies). The TB is also used for subcutaneous injections when a small amount of medication, less than 1 cc, is ordered (e.g., in pediatrics). The TB syringe is calibrated in tenths of a cubic centimeter and in minims and holds only a total of 1 cc, or 1 ml (Fig. 9.9).
3. *Insulin syringe.* Used only for injection of insulin and is calibrated in units. The size in common use today is U-100, in which 100 units of insulin is equal to 1 cc (Fig. 9.10). Formerly insulin and insulin syringes were also available in U-40 and U-80 sizes, and the insulin had to conform to the syringe size. However, these forms are obsolete, and you will be using the U-100 insulin and syringe.

Prefilled cartridges are also available, in which a premeasured amount of a medication is contained in a disposable cartridge with a needle attached. These prefilled units are made ready for injection by placing the cartridge and needle unit in a holder. An example of such a unit is the Carpuject, produced by Winthrop Laboratories, New York (Fig. 9.11). A different type of unit, the Tubex, is produced by Wyeth Laboratories, Philadelphia, Pa.

DRAWING UP MEDICATIONS

1. Wash hands.
2. Assemble equipment (i.e., syringe, needle, packaged alcohol wipes, and medication ampule or vial) on a tray.
3. Check the order using the five Rights of Medication Administration.
4. If medication is contained in a vial, first remove the protective cap. If the vial has been opened previously, wipe the rubber diaphragm on top with

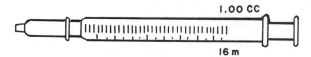

Figure 9.9 *Tuberculin syringe.*

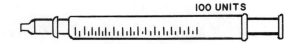

IOO UNITS

Figure 9.10 *Insulin syringe.*

Directions for use of
Carpuject®
Sterile Cartridge-Needle Units

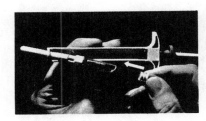

1 Insert CARPUJECT Sterile Cartridge-Needle Unit, needle end first, into open side of holder.

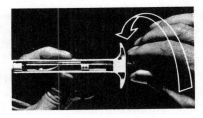

2 Advance and engage blue locking screw and turn *clockwise* beyond initial resistance until it will no longer rotate.

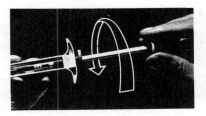

3 Advance plunger rod and screw *clockwise* onto threaded insert in rubber plunger.
To maintain sterility, leave needle guard in place until just before use.

Prepare CARPUJECT unit for administration in a normal manner, ie, remove needle guard, dispel air from cartridge, and proceed with injection.

Figure 9.11 *Carpuject prefilled cartridge. (Reprinted with permission from Winthrop Laboratories, New York.)*

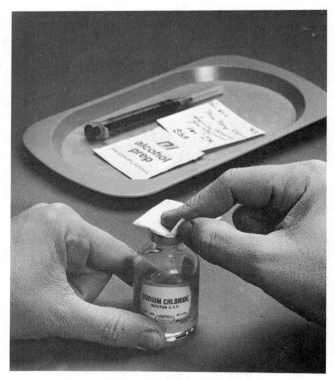

Figure 9.12   *Preparing to withdraw medication from a vial.*

an alcohol wipe. Check vial for date and discoloration of contents (Fig. 9.12).

5. Seat the needle securely on the syringe by pressing firmly downward on the top of the needle cover, and then pull the needle cover straight off.

6. Draw air into the syringe equal to the amount of solution you will be withdrawing from the vial. Insert needle into center of rubber diaphragm and inject air into vial (Fig. 9.13). Invert vial and withdraw prescribed dosage (Fig. 9.14). Be sure syringe is filled to proper level with solution and no bubbles are present.

7. Withdraw needle from vial and replace needle cover carefully without contaminating needle. Brace syringe on side of hand and drop cap over needle. For intramuscular injections, a small bubble (0.2 cc) of air may be added to the syringe *after* the correct dose of medication has been drawn up.

8. If medication is contained in an ampule, hold tip with alcohol wipe to protect your fingers and break open along the scored marking at the neck. Tip vial and withdraw prescribed amount of medication. Recap needle carefully (Fig. 9.15).

9. Place filled syringe with needle covered on tray with alcohol wipes and patient's name card.

☞ *If two drugs are to be combined in a syringe, you must first check for compatibility of the drugs.*

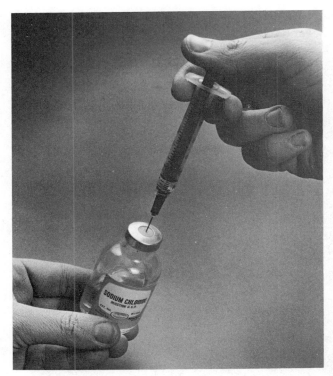

Figure 9.13 *Injection of air into vial.*

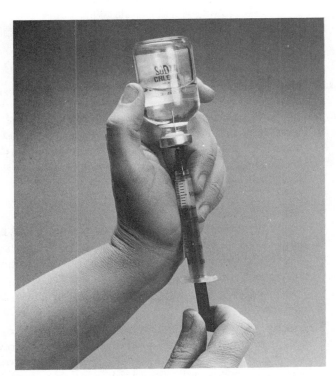

Figure 9.14 *Withdrawal of prescribed amount of medication.*

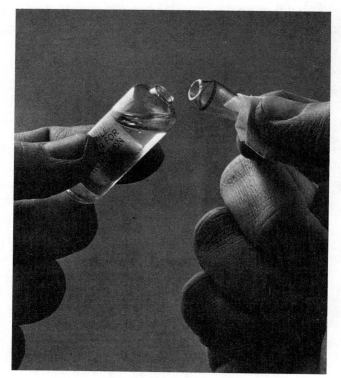

Figure 9.15 *Careful breaking of ampule.*

ADMINISTRATION BY INJECTION

Intradermal injections are usually administered into the skin on the inner surface of the lower arm. For allergy testing, the upper chest and upper back areas may also be used. A small amount (0.1–0.2 ml) is injected so close to the surface that a wheal, or bubble, is formed by the skin expanding (Fig. 9.16).

Technique for intradermal injection is as follows:

1. Wash hands.
2. Assemble equipment (i.e., TB syringe, 26 or 27 gauge, ⅜-inch needle, alcohol wipes, and medication).
3. Check the order using the five Rights of Medication Administration and draw up medication.
4. Identify patient and explain procedure. Arm should be supported on flat surface.
5. Cleanse skin with alcohol wipe on inner surface of the forearm (or other area if ordered by the physician). Allow the skin to dry thoroughly. (If you inject before the skin is dry, you might introduce alcohol into the skin and interfere with test results). Avoid areas with hair or blemishes.
6. Hold the patient's arm in your nondominant hand and stretch the skin taut.

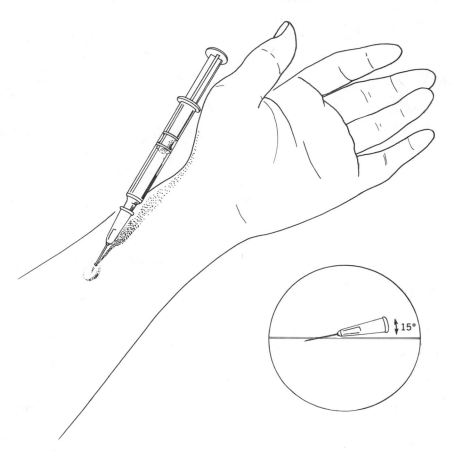

Figure 9.16 *Intradermal injection.*

7. Hold the syringe so that the bevel is up and the needle almost flat against the patient's arm. Insert the needle slowly only far enough to cover the lumen or opening in the needle. The point of the needle should be visible through the skin.

8. Inject the medication *very slowly*. You should see a small white bubble in the skin begin forming immediately. If no bubble forms, withdraw the needle slightly; it may be too deep. If solution leaks out as you inject, the needle is not deep enough.

9. After correct amount of medication is injected, withdraw needle and apply gentle pressure with alcohol wipe. *Do not* massage the area or you may interfere with test results.

10. Note drug name, dosage, time, date, and site of injection on patient's record.

11. Instruct the patient not to scrub, scratch, or rub the area. Provide written instructions regarding time to return for reading. Tell the patient to contact the physician immediately or report to an emergency facility if breathing difficulty, hives, or a rash appears.

☞ *Caution: do not start allergy testing unless emergency equipment is available nearby and personnel are trained in emergency care in case of anaphylactic response.*

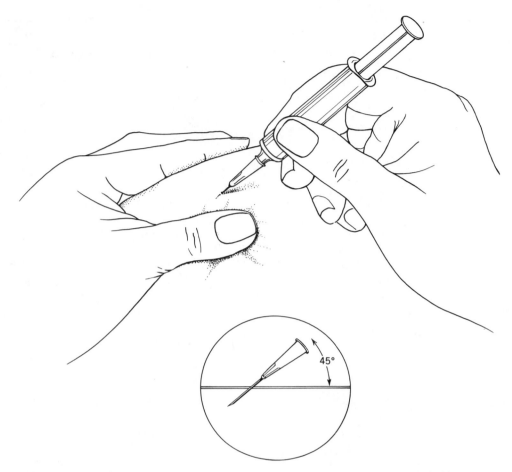

Figure 9.17 *Subcutaneous injection. The tissue is pinched, and the needle is held at a 45-degree angle.*

Subcutaneous injections are administered into the fatty tissues on the upper outer arm, front of the thigh, abdomen, or upper back (Fig. 9.17). A 2½–3-cc syringe is usually used with a 24–26-gauge, ⅜–⅝-inch needle. No more than 2 cc of medication may be administered subcutaneously.

Technique for subcutaneous injection is as follows:

1. Wash hands.
2. Assemble equipment (correct-size syringe and needle, alcohol wipes, and medication).
3. Check the order with the five Rights of Medication Administration and draw up medication.
4. Identify patient and explain procedure.
5. If patient is receiving frequent injections, be sure to rotate injection sites.
6. Cleanse skin with alcohol wipe.
7. Pinch the skin into a fat fold of at least 1 inch (Fig. 9.17).
8. Insert the needle at a 45-degree angle. Then release skin fold.
9. Pull back on the plunger (aspirate). If any blood appears in the syringe,

withdraw the needle. Change to another sterile needle, and replace solution if it is also discolored. Then try a new site for injection.

10. Inject the medication *slowly*, pushing the plunger all the way. Too rapid injection may cause pain.

11. Place alcohol wipe over the entry site, applying pressure with it, as you withdraw the needle.

12. Massage the site gently with the alcohol wipe to speed absorption. (*Do not* massage with heparin injection.) Be sure there is no bleeding.

13. Recap the needle *carefully* for safety. (Follow policy of the facility.)

14. Remove and dispose of all equipment in container provided. Be sure that syringes and needles are handled according to policy at your facility. The Communicable Disease Center now recommends that used needles should *not* be recapped, but should be placed immediately in a puncture-proof container (Sharps box) to prevent the spread of infection.

15. Note the medication, dosage, time, date, site of injection, and your signature on the patient's record.

16. Observe the patient for effects and record observations.

Intramuscular injections are administered deep into large muscles (Fig. 9.18). There are five recommended sites:

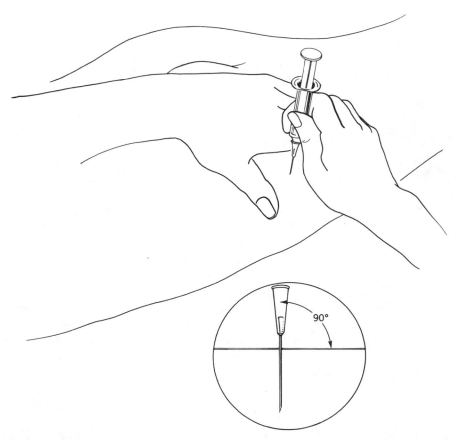

Figure 9.18 *Intramuscular injection. The skin is held taut, with the needle at a 90-degree angle.*

1. *Dorsogluteal.* Upper outer quadrant of the buttock.
2. *Ventrogluteal.* Above and to the outside of the buttock area.
3. *Deltoid.* Upper outer arm above the axilla.
4. *Vastus lateralis.* Front of the thigh toward the outside of the leg.
5. *Rectus femoris.* Front of the thigh toward the midline of the leg.

The intramuscular route has two advantages over the subcutaneous route:

1. A larger amount of solution can be administered (up to 3 cc, or a maximum of 1 cc in children).
2. Absorption is more rapid because the muscle tissue is more vascular (i.e., contains many blood vessels).

The needle must be long enough to go through the subcutaneous tissue into the muscle. The length of the needle varies with the size of the patient. With a child or very thin, emaciated adult, a 1-inch needle is usually adequate. For most adults, a 1½-inch needle is appropriate. However, for an obese person, a 2-inch needle might be required. The needle is inserted at a 90-degree angle with the skin spread taut (Fig. 9.18).

Because there are more large blood vessels and nerves in this deeper tissue, the site for injection must be chosen more precisely. Using the illustrations as a guide, follow these steps in selecting the site:

1. *Dorsogluteal site.* Most commonly used for adults, but not for children under 3 years old (Fig. 9.19). Position the patient flat on the stomach (prone) with the toes pointed inward or on the side with the upper leg flexed. Identify the site by drawing an imaginary line from the posterior superior iliac spine to the greater trochanter of the femur. These two bony prominences can be palpated with the thumb and forefinger. The injection is given above and to the outside of this line. Note that this site is high enough to avoid the sciatic nerve and the major blood vessels.
2. *Ventrogluteal site.* Can be used for all patients. Position the patient on the back or side (Fig. 9.20). Identify the site by placing the palm of your hand on the patient's greater trochanter. Place the index finger on the anterior superior iliac spine and the middle finger on the iliac crest. The injection is made into the center of the V formed between the index and middle fingers.
3. *Deltoid site.* Seldom used because the muscle is smaller and is close to the radial nerve (Fig. 9.21). The maximum solution that can be used is 1 cc; and a shorter needle, 1 inch, is used. Caution must be exercised to avoid the clavicle, humerus, acromium, brachial vein and artery, and radial nerve. Identify the site by drawing an imaginary line across the arm at the level of the armpit. The injection is made above this line and below the acromium on the outer aspect of the arm.
4. *Vastus lateralis.* Located on the anterior lateral thigh, the preferred site for infants, since these muscles are the most developed for children under the age of 3 years (Fig. 9.22). In the elderly, nonambulatory, and emaciated adult, this muscle may be wasted and insufficient for injection. Identify the midportion on the side of the thigh by measuring one hand breadth above the knee and one hand breadth below the great trochanter. The area between is the site for injection.

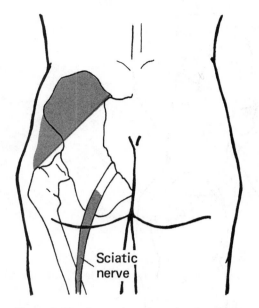

Figure 9.19 Dorsogluteal site for IM injection.

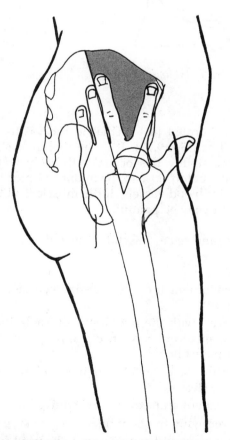

Figure 9.20 Ventrogluteal site for IM injection.

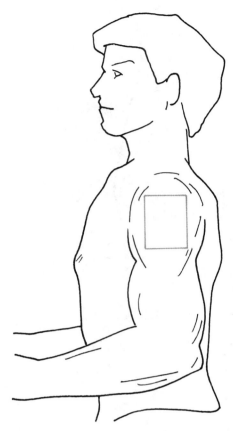

Figure 9.21 *Deltoid site for IM injection.*

5. *Rectus femoris.* Located just medial to the vastus lateralis, but does not cross the midline (Fig. 9.23). It is the preferred site for self-injection because of its accessibility. It is located in the same way as the vastus lateralis. *Caution:* do not get too close to the midline, which is adjacent to the sciatic nerve and major blood vessels. If the muscle is not well developed, injections in this site may be painful.

Technique for intramuscular injection is as follows:

1. Wash hands.
2. Assemble equipment (i.e., correct-size syringe, needle, alcohol wipes, and medication).
3. Check the order with the five Rights of Medication Administration and draw up the medication or insert appropriate prefilled cartridge into Tubex or Carpuject holder.
4. After measuring correct amount of medication in syringe, draw 0.2 cc air into syringe to clear needle.
5. Identify the patient and explain procedure.
6. If patient is receiving frequent injections, be sure to rotate sites.
7. Position the patient and expose area to be used for injection.

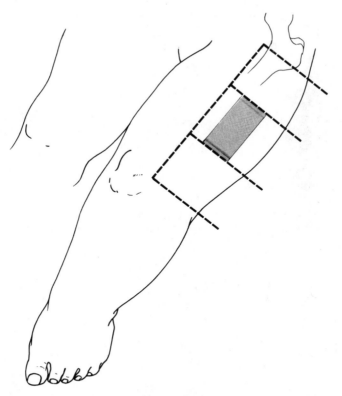

Figure 9.22 *Vastus lateralis site for IM injection, preferred for infants.*

8. Cleanse skin with alcohol wipe.
9. With your nondominant hand, stretch the skin taut at the injection site.
10. Insert the needle at a 90-degree angle with a quick dartlike motion of your dominant hand.
11. Pull back on the plunger (aspirate), and follow previous guidelines if blood appears.
12. Inject the medication at a slow, even rate.
13. Withdraw the needle rapidly.
14. Apply pressure and massage area gently with alcohol wipe.
    Do not massage area if medication is irritating (e.g., hydroxyzine (Vistaril); just apply pressure. Be sure there is no bleeding.
15. Recap the needle carefully. (Follow policy of the facility.)
16. Remove and dispose of all equipment in container provided according to rules of the facility.
17. Note the medication, dosage, time, date, site of injection, and your signature on the patient's record.
18. Observe the patient for effects and record observations.

The *Z-track method* (Fig. 9.24) is used for injections that are irritating to the tissue, such as iron dextran (Imferon). The dorsogluteal is the site for this type of intramuscular injection.

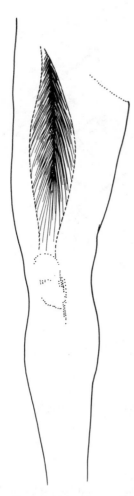

Figure 9.23 *Rectus femoris site for IM injection.*

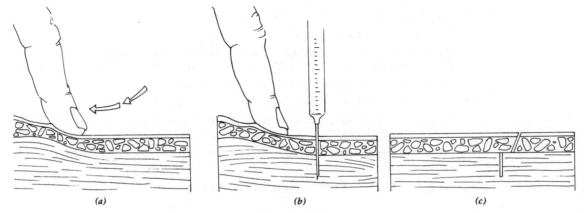

(a)   (b)   (c)

Figure 9.24 *Z-track method of IM injection of iron preparations. (a) Skin and subcutaneous tissue pulled to one side and held there. (b) Needle in place in muscle. (c) Z-track sealed when tissue released.*

Technique for the Z-track method is as follows:

1. Draw up the medication and then add 0.3–0.5 cc of air to the syringe. Then replace the needle with a sterile one 2–3 inches long.
2. Stretch the skin as far as you can to the outer side and hold it there.
3. After cleansing the site, insert the needle with a dartlike motion, aspirate, and then inject the medication *slowly.* Wait 10 sec before withdrawing the needle.
4. Withdraw the needle and allow the skin to return to normal position. This seals off the needle track.
5. *Do not* massage the site, as this could spread the medication to the subcutaneous tissue, causing irritation.
6. Advise the patient that walking will aid absorption and to avoid tight garments, such as girdles, that cause pressure on the site.

Skin Medications

Topical medications for the skin are prescribed for a great variety of conditions and are available in a variety of forms: ointments, lotions, creams, solutions, soaks, and baths. Administration of topical medications requires knowledge of the condition being treated and the purpose of the treatment, and strict adherence to directions as prescribed by the doctor or provided by the pharmacist, or to instructions on the medication container or in a package insert. *When in doubt regarding administration techniques, always ask* a qualified person for advice. Some specific principles for skin medications are outlined in Chapter 12. In addition, good judgment is also required.

Several suggestions for applying topical medication include:

1. For burns, use sterile gloves to apply and cover with sterile dressings because of the danger of infection. Use gentle, light touch because of pain.
2. For skin conditions in which there is irritation or itching, use cotton or snug-fitting gloves to apply. *Never* use gauze, which can cause additional irritation and discomfort.
3. Follow physician's order regarding covering or leaving open to the air.
4. Wash old medication off before applying new, unless specifically directed to do otherwise.

Application to the Mucous Membranes

Medications applied to the mucous membranes also come in a variety of forms: suppositories, ointments, solutions, sprays, gargles, and so on. Always follow the specific directions that accompany the individual medication, unless directed to do otherwise by the physician.

Eye Medications

Instillation of eye medications is described in Chapter 14.

When in doubt about administration of any medication, always ask a qualified person for advice. Never guess! Remember that the patient who is receiving the medication could be you or your loved one. By thinking of yourself in the patient's place you will have the proper attitude to administer medications with competence, good judgment, and compassion.

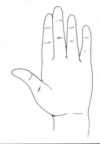

STOP!
Check your knowledge of this chapter before going any further.

CHECKLIST FOR INTRADERMAL INJECTION

ACTIVITY	RATING	
	S	**U**
1. Washed hands.		
2. Checked medication order for date, dosage, time, route, and allergies.		
3. Identified medication: purpose, side effects, cautions, and normal dosage range.		
4. Assembled supplies: TB syringe; 27-gauge, ⅜-inch needle; alcohol wipes; and medication, placed on tray with patient identification card.		
5. Checked medication vial against medication sheet using the five Rights of Medication Administration.		
6. Withdrew correct dose from vial *after* cleansing top with alcohol and injecting equivalent amount of air into vial.		
7. Recapped needle using sterile technique.		
8. Identified patient by checking bracelet and calling patient by name.		
9. Explained procedure to patient and answered any questions regarding procedure.		
10. Positioned patient with inner forearm exposed and supported on a flat surface.		
11. Selected area without hair or blemish, cleansed skin with alcohol wipe, and allowed skin to dry.		
12. Held patient's arm with nondominant hand, stretching the skin taut.		
13. Expelled any air bubbles from syringe.		
14. Inserted needle point slowly, only enough to cover needle opening. Point of needle visible through skin.		
15. Injected medication very slowly with immediate formation of small bleb.		
16. Withdrew needle and applied gentle pressure to injection site with alcohol wipe (no massage).		
17. Recorded drug name, dosage, time, date, and site of injection on patient's record and signed or initialed entry.		
18. Disposed of syringe and needle in correct place, according to policy of facility.		
19. Observed patient for 30 min for possible anaphylactic reaction. Identified location of emergency equipment and medication if required.		
20. Provided written instructions regarding time to return for reading. Instructed patient to avoid scrubbing, scratching, or rubbing the area and to report to emergency facility with dyspnea, hives, or rash.		

Note: s, satisfactory; u, unsatisfactory.

CHECKLIST FOR SUBCUTANEOUS INJECTION

ACTIVITY	RATING	
	S	**U**
1. Washed hands.		
2. Checked medication order for date, dosage, time, route, and allergies.		
3. Identified medication: purpose, side effects, contraindications, interactions, and normal dosage range.		
4. Assembled supplies: 2½–3-cc, TB or insulin syringe; 24–26 gauge, ⅜–⅝ inch needle; alcohol wipes; and medication vial or ampoule on tray with patient identification card.		
5. Checked medication against medication sheet using the five Rights of Medication Administration. Also checked drug for date and discoloration.		
6. Calculated correct dosage on paper if necessary and checked calculations with instructor.		
7. If drug contained in *vial*, withdrew correct amount after cleansing top with alcohol wipe and injecting equivalent amount of air into vial. If drug contained in *ampule*, held tip with alcohol wipe while breaking it at neck. Withdrew correct amount of drug without bubbles in syringe.		
8. Recapped needle using sterile technique and placed filled syringe on tray with supplies.		
9. Identified patient by checking identification bracelet and calling patient by name.		
10. Explained procedure to patient and answered any questions.		
11. Selected appropriate site, using rotation if frequent injections.		
12. Cleansed skin with alcohol wipe.		
13. Pinched skin into fold with nondominant hand.		
14. Expelled any air bubbles from syringe.		
15. Inserted needle at a 45-degree angle and released skin fold.		
16. While holding needle hub with nondominant hand, aspirated for blood (used new site if necessary).		
17. Injected medication slowly.		
18. Placed alcohol wipe over entry site, and applied pressure as needle was withdrawn. Massaged site gently (with heparin, pressure only, no massage.)		
19. Disposed of syringe and needle in correct place, according to policy of the facility.		
20. Recorded drug, name, dosage, time, date, site of injection, and signature on patient's record.		

Note: s, satisfactory; u, unsatisfactory.

CHECKLIST FOR INTRAMUSCULAR INJECTION

ACTIVITY	RATING	
	S	U
1. Washed hands.		
2. Checked medication order for date, dosage, time, route, and allergies.		
3. Identified medication: purpose, side effects, cautions, and normal dosage range.		
4. Assembled supplies: 2½–3-cc Tubex or Carpuject syringe; 1½–2 inch needle, usually 21 gauge; alcohol wipes; and medication on tray with patient identification card.		
5. Checked medication against medication sheet using the five Rights of Medication Administration. If PRN medication, checked time of last dose.		
6. Calculated correct dosage on paper if necessary, and checked time of last dose.		
7. If drug contained in *vial*, withdrew correct amount after cleansing top with alcohol wipe and injecting equivalent amount of air into vial. If drug contained in *ampoule*, held tip with alcohol wipe while breaking it at neck. Withdrew correct amount of drug without bubbles in syringe. If drug contained in cartridge, assembled correctly in holder with drug at right level for dosage and no bubbles in syringe.		
8. *After* drug measured accurately in syringe, drew 0.2 cc air into syringe.		
9. Recapped needle using sterile technique, and placed filled syringe on tray with supplies.		
10. Identified patient by checking bracelet and calling patient by name.		
11. Explained procedure to patient and answered any questions.		
12. Closed door to room and/or curtain around bed.		
13. Selected appropriate site, using rotation if frequent injections.		
14. Positioned patient appropriately, exposing only the area for injection.		
15. Cleansed skin with alcohol wipe.		
16. With forefinger and thumb of nondominant hand, spread the skin taut at injection site.		
17. Inserted needle at a 90-degree angle with a quick, dartlike motion of dominant hand.		
18. Aspirated for blood (used new site if necessary).		
19. Injected medication at a slow, even rate.		
20. Applied pressure with alcohol wipe over entry site as needle was withdrawn rapidly. Massaged site gently with alcohol wipe unless medication irritating (with Ancef, Vistaril, or Imferon, pressure only, no massage).		

Note: s, satisfactory; u, unsatisfactory.

CHECKLIST FOR INTRAMUSCULAR INJECTION

ACTIVITY	RATING	
	S	**U**
21. Made sure there was no bleeding before covering patient and making patient comfortable.		
22. Disposed of syringe and needle in correct place, according to policy of facility.		
23. Recorded drug, name, dosage, time, date, site of injection, and signature on patient's record.		

Note: s, satisfactory; u, unsatisfactory.

CHAPTER REVIEW QUIZ

Fill in the blanks:

1. Parenteral includes any routes other than

_____ .

2. Systemic effects are those affecting _____ .

3. The four parenteral routes with systemic effects include:

_____   _____

_____   _____

Label the routes according to their action. Use R for rapid and S for slow. Match each route with the appropriate definition:

	Action			Definition
4.	_____	Sublingual	_____	a. Given with a needle
5.	_____	Transcutaneous	_____	b. Nebulizer or IPPB
6.	_____	Inhalation	_____	c. Under the tongue
7.	_____	Injection	_____	d. Skin patch

8. What precaution should be observed when applying transcutaneous systems?

9. IPPB refers to _____ .

Select the correct needle for the purpose. Needle size may be used for more than one purpose:

	Purpose		Needle
10.	_____	Subcutaneous injection	a. 21 gauge, 1½ inch
11.	_____	Intravenous injection	b. 25 gauge, ⅝ inch
12.	_____	Allergy testing	c. 18 gauge
13.	_____	Intramuscular injection	d. 27 gauge, ⅜ inch

14. What are the two purposes of the tuberculin syringe?

_____

_____

15. The insulin syringe is calibrated in _____ ,
and 1 cc is equal to _____
in an insulin syringe.

16. Disposable cartridges containing a premeasured amount of medication
are used with a white plastic holder called a _____
or a metal holder called a _____ .

Match the injection with the proper technique:

	Injection		Technique
17.	____ Intramuscular	a.	Needle 45-degree angle, skin pinched up
18.	____ Subcutaneous	b.	Needle flat, bevel up, skin taut
19.	____ Intradermal	c.	Needle 90-degree angle, skin taut

20. List the five sites for intramuscular injections and when each is used.

_____   _____

_____   _____

_____   _____

_____   _____

_____   _____

21. Why is the Z-track method used? _____
Describe Z-track administration. _____

_____

_____

_____

22. Define local effects. _____
List four areas to administer medication for local effects.

_____

_____

_____

_____

10

Poison Control

OBJECTIVES

Upon completion of this chapter, the student will be able to:

1. Define poison, overdose, emetic, antidote, and ingestion.
2. Identify four routes by which poisons may be taken into the body.
3. List four conditions in which an emetic would not be given to induce vomiting, and describe substitute therapy to remove poison.
4. Describe medication, dosage, and procedure for administration of the most common emetic.
5. Explain the purpose of activated charcoal and when it is given.
6. Name three clinical procedures required when caring for patients who have been poisoned.
7. Describe appropriate therapy for poisoning by inhalation, external poison, insect sting, and snakebite.
8. Identify two groups of people at risk for poisoning.
9. List ten recommendations for patient education to help prevent poisoning.

A poison is a substance taken into the body by ingestion, inhalation, injection or absorption that interferes with normal physiological functions. In some cases, only a small amount of a substance can cause severe tissue damage directly (e.g., corrosives). In other cases, the substance can be beneficial in small amounts, but lethal in excessive amounts (e.g., overdose of a medication).

In a case of suspected poisoning, the best policy is to contact a Poison Control Center through an emergency care facility. Instructions can then be given by phone for appropriate emergency treatment based on the type of poison and the patient's condition, age, and size.

Poisoning by Ingestion

The most common type of poisoning is by ingestion, or swallowing. An emetic, such as ipecac syrup, is usually administered to induce vomiting. However, there are some important exceptions to this therapy. *Do not* induce vomiting under these conditions:

1. Ingestion of corrosive substances such as mineral acids or caustic alkalis (e.g., cabolic acid, ammonia, and lye). Vomiting can cause additional tissue damage.
2. Ingestion of volatile petroleum products (e.g., gasoline, kerosene, lighter fluid, and benzene). Vomiting can cause aspiration and/or asphyxiation.
3. Ingestion of convulsants (e.g., strychnine or iodine). Vomiting can precipitate seizures.
4. If patient is semiconscious, severely inebriated, in shock, or has no gag reflex. Vomiting could cause choking, aspiration, and/or asphyxiation.

Caution must be taken with the use of ipecac in patients with cardiac or vascular disease. Vomiting can increase blood pressure and precipitate a stroke, cardiac arrhythmias, or atrioventricular block.

If any of the abovementioned conditions exists, the patient should be transported *immediately* to an emergency care facility. Trained personnel can remove the stomach contents by gastric lavage and administer appropriate antidotes as indicated.

Antidotes, such as CNS stimulants and/or CPR, may be required in poisoning with CNS depressants. Gastric lavage is *not* used in patients who have ingested corrosives, because of the danger of perforating the damaged tissue of the esophagus. If perforation exists, surgery is required. Observation is required in an acute care facility.

If none of the abovementioned conditions exists and the patient is able to swallow, 15–30 ml of ipecac syrup is administered PO and followed immediately with several glasses (at least 1 qt) of water. Other liquids may be substituted for water. However, milk may slow emesis and carbonated drinks may cause distention; these liquids should therefore be avoided. If emesis does not occur within 20 min, the initial dose of 15 ml may be repeated. If there is no emesis within 30 min, gastric lavage is required.

Sometimes a substance such as activated charcoal is administered to minimize systemic absorption of the ingested poison. However, activated charcoal is given *only after* emesis or gastric lavage. If given before the ipecac, it will absorb the ipecac and prevent emesis.

Personnel caring for poisoning victims should observe the following cautions:

- Be sure to save emesis. It may be necessary to send it to a laboratory to determine the type of poison. If there is doubt about the poison, the doctor may also order urine and blood tests for toxicology.
- Closely monitor the vital signs of patients who have taken poison of any kind.
- Observe closely for possible confusion, tremors, convulsions, visual disturbances, loss of consciousness, respiratory distress, or cardiac arrhythmias.

Poisoning by Inhalation

Poisoning by inhalation requires symptomatic treatment: fresh air, oxygen, and CPR if indicated. Inhaling insect spray may require administration of an antidote.

External Poisoning

External poisons should be flushed from the skin or eyes with a continuous stream of water. The patient should then be transported to an emergency care facility for further treatment as required. Systemic absorption of poisons through the skin may require administration of an antidote.

Poisoning by Insect Sting and Snakebite

Poisoning by insect sting (e.g., bee, wasp, scorpion, or fire ant) should be treated with an ice pack. If the patient is allergic, watch closely for possible anaphylactic reaction. CPR and administration of adrenalin and corticosteroids may be required. Transport the patient to an emergency care facility immediately if indicated. Some allergic persons carry a kit with medication prescribed by their doctor (e.g., antihistamine and Isuprel SL to be self-administered if stung, or epinephrine for self-injection or injection by someone else).

Do not apply ice or tourniquet to snakebite. Venom is very irritating and may cause sloughing of the tissues. Keep the patient quiet in order to slow circulation, and transport the patient, lying down, to an emergency care facility for antivenom injections.

PATIENT EDUCATION

Public education is of paramount importance in preventing poisoning. The general public must be instructed in precautions with medications, and it is especially important to inform the parents and caretakers of young children, and the elderly. It is the responsibility of all health care workers to provide the necessary information to help prevent poisoning.

To prevent poisoning, the American Medical Association recommends the following precautions:

1. Keep all medicines, household chemicals, and other substances in a locked cupboard. There is no place that is "out of reach of children."
2. Never transfer poisonous substances to unlabeled containers or to food containers such as milk or soda bottles or cereal boxes.
3. Never store poisonous substances in the same area with food. Confusion could be fatal.
4. Never reuse containers of chemical products.
5. When discarding medication, always flush down the toilet. Never discard it in wastebasket.
6. Do not give or take medications in the dark.
7. Never leave medications on a bedside stand. Confusion while a person is sleepy could result in a fatal overdose.
8. Always read the label before taking any medication or pouring any solution for ingestion.
9. Never tell children the medicine you are giving them is candy.
10. When preparing a baby's formula, taste the ingredients. Never store boric acid, salt, or talcum near the formula ingredients.
11. Never give or take any medication that is discolored, has a strange odor, or is outdated.

Questions concerning poisons and appropriate treatment for poisoning can be referred to any emergency care facility. There are also more than 500 Poison Control Centers throughout the United States with computerized data to further assist you in obtaining information about poisons.

People at Risk

Poisoning is a major cause of death among young children because of their natural curiosity and active life-style. The danger is particularly great with flavored medications, such as aspirin or iron tablets. Great care must be taken to prevent poisoning of young children.

Another group at risk for poisoning is the elderly. Overdoses of medication can result in toxicity, with symptoms of confusion, dizziness, weakness, lethargy, ataxia, tremors, or cardiac irregularities. *Toxic reactions* from medications taken by the elderly can possibly result from:

1. Slower metabolism, impaired circulation, and decreased excretion, causing medication to remain in the body longer and build up to dangerous levels.
2. Wrong dosage due to impaired vision or poor memory (patients may forget that they have taken medicine and take a double dose).

3. Interactions when many different medications are taken and over-the-counter medications are self-administered with inadequate medical supervision.
4. Medical conditions affecting absorption.

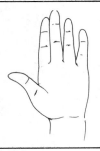

STOP!
Check your knowledge of this chapter before going any further.

CHAPTER REVIEW QUIZ

Complete the statements by filling in the blanks:

1. Poisons can be taken into the body in four different ways:

   _____

   _____

   _____

   _____

2. In cases of poison ingestion, emetics are contraindicated under the following four conditions:

   _____

   _____

   _____

   _____

3. Gastric lavage is contraindicated when a patient has ingested what type of substance?

   _____

4. When is activated charcoal administered?

   _____

5. Why are gastric contents saved after emesis or gastric lavage?

   _____

6. What is the treatment for poisons that contact skin or eyes?

   _____

   _____

7. What two groups of people are most at risk for poisoning?

   _____

   _____

8. Name four conditions that may cause toxic medication reactions in the elderly.

   _____

   _____

   _____

   _____

COMPREHENSIVE REVIEW EXAM FOR PART I

1. Drug standards regulate all of the following factors in drug preparation *except:*

   a. strength
   b. purity
   c. color
   d. quality

2. All of the following facts are true of the Pure Food and Drug Act *except:*

   a. for consumer protection
   b. listed approved drugs
   c. set minimal standards
   d. passed in 1776

3. The Food and Drug Administration regulates all of the following drug factors *except:*

   a. prescription labeling
   b. shape of tablet
   c. effectiveness
   d. safety

4. Which of the following drugs is *not* a controlled substance?

   a. marijuana
   b. Valium
   c. codeine
   d. thyroid

5. Which statement is *not* true of controlled drugs?

   a. listed by schedule
   b. refilled PRN
   c. may cause dependence
   d. sometimes illegal

6. Which is *not* a good source of drug information?

   a. PDR
   b. USP/NF
   c. drug insert
   d. news magazine

7. Which statement is true of the generic name of a drug?

   a. assigned by drug company
   b. written in capital letters
   c. common name
   d. same as trade name

8. The term OTC refers to drugs:

   a. oftentimes controlled
   b. requiring prescription
   c. for sale to anyone
   d. officially certified

9. Which of the following conditions is *not* commonly listed as a *contraindication* for drug administration?

   a. obesity
   b. allergy
   c. pregnancy
   d. lactation

10. Before giving a new drug, you must know all of the following *except:*

a. interactions   c. side effects
b. contraindications   d. usual price

11. An antibiotic with *photosensitivity* listed as a side effect could causes:

a. deafness   c. blindness
b. sunburn   d. kidney damage

12. Which is *not* a source of drugs?

a. minerals   c. animals
b. gases   d. laboratory

13. Which is *not* a process that drugs go through in the body?

a. tolerance   c. metabolism
b. distribution   d. excretion

14. Which of the following patient characteristics is *not* a factor affecting the processing of drugs in the body?

a. weight   c. mental state
b. age   d. skin color

15. Drug toxicity from cumulative effects may result from all of the following *except:*

a. low metabolism   c. high blood pressure
b. poor circulation   d. kidney malfunction

16. Which term does *not* describe an adverse or unexpected result from a drug?

a. idiosyncracy   c. placebo effect
b. anaphylaxis   d. teratogenic effect

17. Which route of administration is used most often?

a. topical   c. injection
b. sublingual   d. oral

18. Which is *not* a form of parenteral administration?

a. inhalation   c. dermal patch
b. rectal   d. injection

19. Which type of medication can be crushed and mixed with food to facilitate administration?

a. timed-release capsule   c. scored tablet
b. lozenge   d. enteric-coated tablet

20. Which is *not* a topical form of administration?

a. ointment   c. eye drops
b. intradermal   d. vaginal cream

21. Which is the most rapid form of administration?

a. PO

b. IV

c. IM

d. SC

22. Which is the least accurate system for measuring medication?

a. metric

b. apothecary

c. household

23. Which is the most frequently used system for measuring medicine?

a. apothecary

b. metric

c. household

24. Medication orders must contain all of the following *except:*

a. dosage

b. route

c. medication name

d. patient's address

25. The prescription blank for a controlled substance must contain all of the following *except:*

a. physician's DEA number

b. generic name

c. frequency

d. number of refills

26. Which type of equipment is *least* accurate in measuring medicine?

a. medicine cup

b. minim glass

c. teaspoon

d. syringe

27. Responsibilities of the health care worker include all of the following *except:*

a. patient education

b. current information

c. judgment

d. prescribing

28. Which is *not* appropriate action after administration of medication?

a. assessment

b. research concerning meals

c. evaluation

d. documentation

29. Which is the *least* helpful information in dispensing medication?

a. allergies

b. handicaps

c. health history

d. patient's occupation

30. If a medication error is made, all of the following actions are required *except:*

a. report to physician

b. file incident report

c. note on patient record

d. apologize to patient

31. Before giving any medicine, it is essential to review the five Rights of Medication Administration, including all of the following *except:*

a. right amount

b. right drug

c. right drug company

d. right time schedule

32. Documentation of a controlled drug given PRN for pain requires all of the following *except:*

    a. note on narcotic record
    b. note of trade name
    c. note of effectiveness
    d. note on patient record

33. Which one is *not* used for administration by the gastrointestinal route?

    a. nasogastric tube
    b. hand-held nebulizer
    c. rectal suppository
    d. timed-release capsule

34. Which one is *not* an advantage of the oral route over other routes?

    a. speed
    b. safety
    c. economy
    d. convenience

35. If a medication is ordered PO and the patient is NPO, which action is *most* appropriate?

    a. give medication by injection
    b. give medication rectally
    c. omit medication and note on chart
    d. consult the person in charge

36. Oral medications are usually best administered with which fluid?

    a. fruit juice
    b. milk
    c. water
    d. hot tea

37. When preparing cough syrup, which is the most appropriate action?

    a. shake the bottle
    b. dilute with liquid
    c. hold label side down
    d. hold medicine cup at eye level

38. Which of the following is *not* required for administration of rectal suppository?

    a. lubricant
    b. privacy
    c. bed elevated
    d. finger cot

39. Which parenteral route is not usually administered for systemic effects?

    a. transdermal
    b. topical
    c. sublingual
    d. inhalation

40. Which route has the slowest action?

    a. transcutaneous
    b. inhalation
    c. sublingual
    d. injection

41. Which is *not* a form of inhalation therapy?

    a. Whirlybird Spinhaler
    b. metered-dose nebulizer
    c. IPPB
    d. otic drops

42. Which is *not* appropriate for intradermal injection?

    a. tuberculin syringe
    b. 21-gauge, 1-inch needle
    c. wheal formation on skin
    d. 0.1–0.2 ml solution

43. Which is *not* true of intramuscular injections?

a. skin held taut

b. 1½-inch needle usual

c. 45-degree angle of needle

d. can be Z track

44. Which one of these intramuscular injection sites is used for infants?

a. dorsogluteal

b. ventrogluteal

c. deltoid

d. vastus lateralis

45. Ipecac to induce vomiting would be indicated in poisoning with which substance?

a. ammonia

b. strychnine

c. lighter fluid

d. aspirin

46. Ipecac would be contraindicated in patients with all of the following conditions *except:*

a. semiconscious

b. hypertension

c. diabetes

d. cardiac

47. If there is doubt about the type of poison, toxicology tests will be done on all of the following *except:*

a. urine

b. stool

c. blood

d. emesis

48. Which group is *least* at risk of accidental poisoning?

a. infants

b. elderly

c. young adults

49. Patient education to prevent poisoning includes all of the following advice *except:*

a. label all medications and poisons

b. discard medications in toilet

c. always read medicine labels

d. keep medications at bedside

Calculate the correct dosage for administration in the following problems. Label your answers. Remember that syringes are not marked in fractions; therefore, when computing dosages for administration, you must convert all fractions to decimals and round off to one decimal place.

50. You are to give 7,500 U of heparin SC. The vial is labeled 10,000 U/ml. How many milliliters should you give?

51. You are to give 10 ml of Phenergan cough syrup with codeine. The bottle is labeled 10.0 mg of codeine in 5 ml of cough syrup. How much codeine should the patient receive in each prescribed dose?

52. The medicine bottle label states that the strength of each tablet in the bottle is 0.25 mg. The physician has ordered that the patient is to receive 0.5 mg. How many tablets should you give?

53. The physician has ordered 20 mg of Demerol to be given. On hand is medication containing 50 mg/cc. How many cubic centimeters should you give?

PART II

Drugs of the Systems

11

Vitamins and Minerals

OBJECTIVES

Upon completion of this chapter, the student will be able to:

1. Categorize vitamins as water soluble or fat soluble.
2. List vitamins and their sources, function, signs of deficiency, and symptoms of overdose if known.
3. Identify vitamins by name as well as letter.
4. List minerals and their sources, function, and signs of deficiency.
5. Identify the chemical symbol for each mineral.
6. Describe conditions that may require vitamin and/or mineral supplements.

The National Research Council of the Food and Nutrition Board has listed U.S. Recommended Dietary Allowances (U.S. RDA) of vitamins and minerals necessary for maintenance of health in the average adult under normal living conditions. This information was published by the National Academy of Sciences, Washington, D.C., in 1980.

Under special circumstances, vitamin and mineral supplements are required for health maintenance. *Indications* for vitamin and mineral supplements include:

Inadequate diet. Due to anorexia, weight-reduction or other special diets, illness, alcoholism, or poor eating habits.

Malabsorption syndromes. Chronic gastrointestinal disorders or surgery that result in chronic diarrhea.

Increased need for certain nutrients. As in pregnancy, lactation (especially iron and calcium), infants under 1 year of age, adolescence, debilitation, illness, unusual physical activity, postmenopausal women (calcium).

Deficiency due to medication interactions. For example potassium deficiency with diuretic use.

It is important to differentiate between water-soluble and fat-soluble vitamins in order to avoid build-up in the body with possible symptoms of overdose. Megadoses of vitamins (more than the RDA) should be taken only if prescribed by a physician and/or approved by the FDA. Remember, the RDA includes the amount from the foods you eat as well as supplements. Research reports have indicated a possibility of damage to tissues with large quantities of vitamins (above RDA), especially those stored in the fat cells of the body.

The Recommended Dietary Allowances listed on the following pages are established for average, normal, healthy adults. Larger amounts are required with certain conditions (e.g., pregnancy, lactation, and some illnesses). Smaller amounts are required for children. However, megadoses should *never* be taken except under the direct supervision of a physician.

Fat-Soluble Vitamins

The fat-soluble vitamins are A, D, E, and K.

VITAMIN A

Vitamin A is processed in the body from the carotene of plants, especially yellow-orange and dark-green, leafy vegetables and dairy products (RDA, 1,000 U/day).

Necessary for:

Proper visual function at night
Normal growth and development
Healing of wounds (sometimes prescribed for acne)

Deficiencies may result from:

Malabsorption of fats or diarrhea
Obstruction of bile
Presence of mineral oil in the intestines
Overcooking of vegetables in an open container (heat and air cause oxidation)
Prolonged infection or fever

Signs of deficiency include:

Night blindness
Slow growth
Dry eyes and skin, pruritis, and photosensitivity
Impaired healing

Symptoms of overdose (hypervitaminosis A) include:

Fatigue and lethargy
Headache and insomnia
Brittle nails and dry skin
Anorexia, nausea, and diarrhea
Yellow or orange skin pigmentation

Caution should be used with impaired renal or hepatic function.

VITAMIN D

Vitamin D is synthesized in the body through the action of sunlight on the skin. Other sources include fish oils and food products fortified with vitamin D, such as milk and cereals (RDA, 200 U/day).

Necessary for:

Regulating the absorption and metabolism of calcium and phosphorus for healthy bones and teeth
Pregnancy and lactation, when it is especially important

Signs of deficiency include:

Poor tooth and bone structure (rickets)
Skeletal deformities
Osteoporosis
Tetany

Symptoms of overdose include:

GI distress, weakness, and headache
Cardiac arrhythmias

Renal dysfunction
Hypercalcemia and convulsions
Fetal disorders of heart and parathyroid

Caution not to exceed the RDA should be used especially with:

Cardiovascular disorders
Kidney diseases
Pregnancy (RDA, 400–500 U/day)

Interactions (overdose may antagonize) may occur with:

Digitalis
Thiazide diuretics

VITAMIN E

Vitamin E is abundant in nature, found especially in cereals, wheat germ, vegetable oils, eggs, meat, and poultry (RDA, 8–10 U/day).

Necessary for normal metabolism; its exact function is still under investigation.

Deficiencies are found in those with:

Malabsorption
Pathologic conditions of liver and pancreas
Premature infants

Signs of deficiency are not firmly established. Research studies of adults are contradictory and controversial. Premature infants may show irritability, edema, or anemia.

Symptoms of overdose are also not clinically proven. However, since vitamin E is fat soluble, the potential for overdose exists, and caution is urged with megadoses of this and other fat-soluble vitamins.

VITAMIN K

Vitamin K is found in green leafy vegetables, alfalfa, meat, and dairy products and is synthesized by intestinal bacteria (RDA 70–140 μg/day).

Necessary for blood clotting.

Deficiencies may result from reduced prothrombin factors in the blood due to:

Insufficient clotting factors in the newborn
Medication interaction (e.g., with Coumadin)

Signs of deficiency include:

Increased clotting time
Petechiae and bruising
Blood in the urine (hematuria)
Blood in the stool (melena)

No symptoms of overdose have been proven. However, it should be noted that vitamin K is fat soluble and *only* effective in control of hemorrhage due to low concentrations of *prothrombin* in the blood. When other clotting factors are involved, vitamin K is ineffective in controlling bleeding.

Vitamin K (Mephyton) is frequently administered at birth (1 mg IM) or to adults (4–40 mg PO, IM, or IV of Mephyton or Synkayvite) for bleeding disorders due to low prothrombin time. It is also administered as an antidote for bleeding due to coumarin therapy.

Water-Soluble Vitamins

The *water-soluble vitamins* include the B-complex vitamins and vitamin C.

VITAMIN B$_1$

Vitamin B$_1$ (thiamine) is a coenzyme utilized for carbohydrate metabolism. It is found in whole grains, peas, beans, nuts, and enriched cereals (RDA 1–1.4 mg/day).

Necessary for normal function of the nervous and cardiovascular systems.

Deficiencies in the United States may be due to:

Chronic alcoholism
Malabsorption

Signs of deficiency (beriberi) include:

Anorexia and constipation
Neuritis, pain, or tingling in extremities
Muscle weakness, fatigue, and ataxia
Mental depression and memory loss
Heart failure and edema

VITAMIN B$_2$

Vitamin B$_2$ (riboflavin) is a coenzyme utilized in the metabolism of all cells. It is found in milk, dairy products, meats, yeast, and green leafy vegetables (RDA, 1.8 mg/day).

Necessary for cell growth and metabolism.

Deficiencies in the United States may be due to:

Chronic alcoholism
Poor diet during pregnancy

Signs of deficiency include:

Glossitis (inflammation of the tongue)
Cheilosis (cracking at corners of mouth)
Dermatitis and photosensitivity

Overdose resulting from megadoses has been shown to cause nerve damage when taken for extended periods of time.

VITAMIN B$_6$

Vitamin B$_6$ (pyridoxine) is a coenzyme utilized in the metabolism of carbohydrates, fats, and protein. It is found in meats, bananas, potatoes, lima beans, and whole grain cereals (RDA, 2.0–2.2 mg/day).

Deficiencies may be due to:

Chronic alcoholism
Drug interactions with isoniazid, other antitubercular drugs, or oral contraceptives
Cirrhosis
Malabsorption syndromes
Congestive heart failure

Signs of deficiency include:

In infants, seizure activity
In adults, peripheral neuropathy, oral sores, decreased mental function, skin problems, and anemia

Caution: overdose in pregnant women may result in newborns with seizures who have developed a need for greater than normal amounts of pyridoxine.

PATIENT EDUCATION

Patients taking levodopa alone (not combined with carbidopa) should be instructed not to take a vitamin B$_6$ supplement because it antagonizes the action of levodopa.

VITAMIN B$_{12}$

Vitamin B$_{12}$ (cyanocobalamin) is found in meats (especially organ meats), fish, milk, cheese, and eggs. Absorption of vitamin B$_{12}$ depends on an intrinsic factor normally present in the gastric juice of humans. Absence of this factor leads to vitamin B$_{12}$ deficiency and pernicious anemia (RDA, 3 µg/day).

Necessary for maturation of red blood cells.

Deficiencies are associated with:

Vegetarian diets
Gastrectomy or intestinal resections
Malabsorption
Pernicious anemia
Kidney or liver disease

Signs of deficiency include:

Poor muscular coordination
Numbness of hands and feet
Mental confusion and irritability
Anemia and weakness

Treatment for pernicious anemia consists of vitamin B$_{12}$ (Betalin 12 or Rubramin), 100–1,000 µg IM monthly for life.

Side effects include:

Transient diarrhea
Itching and urticaria
Anaphylaxis (rare)

Interactions may occur (decreased absorption of B$_{12}$) with:

Aminoglycoside antibiotics
Anticonvulsants
Slow-release potassium and colchicine

PATIENT EDUCATION

Patients should avoid taking large doses without confirmed deficiency, as megadoses may mask symptoms of folic acid deficiency) or cause complications in those with cardiac or gout conditions.

FOLIC ACID

Folic acid is a vitamin included in the B-complex group and found in fresh fruits and vegetables, yeast, and organ meats (RDA, 400 µg/day).

Necessary for protein synthesis and production of red blood cells.

Deficiencies are associated with:

Improper diet
Chronic alcoholism
Liver pathology
Intestinal obstruction
Megaloblastic anemia
Malabsorption

Signs of deficiency include:

Diarrhea
Sore mouth
Irritability

Caution: folic acid (Folvite) should not be given to anyone with undiagnosed anemia, since it may mask the diagnosis of pernicious anemia.

Interactions may occur with:

Phenytoin (Dilantin)
Estrogen (oral contraceptives)

When these drugs are used, folic acid supplements may be required.

PATIENT EDUCATION

Patients should avoid taking folic acid supplements without consulting a physician first.

NIACIN

Niacin (nicotinic acid) is a vitamin included in the B-complex group and found in beef, milk, eggs, fish, and yeast (RDA, 13–18 mg/day).

Necessary for lipid metabolism and nerve functioning, especially in circulation.

Deficiency results in pellagra.

Signs of deficiency include:

Peripheral vascular insufficiency
Dermatitis and varicose ulcers
Diarrhea
Dementia (mental problems)
Mouth sores

Treatment indications (usually as an adjunct with other medications) include:

Many vascular disorders (e.g., vascular spasm, arteriosclerosis, Raynaud's disease, angina, and varicose and decubital ulcers)
Circulatory disturbances of the inner ear
To lower blood lipid levels

Niacin is not used frequently because of serious side effects.

Side effects include:

Postural hypotension
Jaundice
Nausea, diarrhea, vomiting
Increased blood sugar and uric acid
Headache, flushing, and burning sensations

PATIENT EDUCATION

Patients should be instructed regarding possible side effects, especially flushing and a burning sensation, and cautioned to rise slowly from a reclining position.

VITAMIN C

Vitamin C (ascorbic acid) is a water-soluble vitamin found in fresh fruits and vegetables, especially citrus fruits, cantaloupe, tomatoes, cabbage, green peppers, and broccoli. It is unstable when exposed to heat or air or combined with alkaline compounds (e.g., antacids) (RDA, 60 mg/day).

Necessary for cellular metabolism and intracellular substances (collagen), and for normal teeth, gums, and bones. Also required for iron absorption.

Deficiencies are associated with:

Pregnancy and lactation
Diet lacking fresh fruit and vegetables
Alcoholism, infections, trauma, and stress
GI disease
Smoking

Signs of deficiency (scurvy) include:

Muscle weakness
Sore and bleeding mouth and gums
Capillary fragility (petechiae or bruising)
Degenerative changes in bone and connective tissue
Poor healing

Side effects of large doses of vitamin C can include:

Heartburn, abdominal cramps, nausea, and vomiting
Increased uric acid levels, may precipitate gouty arthritis
Increased urinary calcium, may precipitate kidney stone formation

Interactions may occur with:

Aspirin, causing elevated blood levels of aspirin
Barbiturates, tetracyclines, estrogens, oral contraceptives, which may increase requirements for vitamin C
Alcohol and smoking, which may decrease vitamin C level

PATIENT EDUCATION

Patients should be given the following information:

Vitamin C is destroyed by heat and air; therefore, raw fresh fruits and vegetables are best.

Research studies have failed to prove that vitamin C is effective in prevention or treatment of the common cold.

Large quantities of supplemental vitamin C are to be avoided, unless prescribed by a doctor, because of potential side effects, such as gastric irritation, increased uric acid, and urinary calcium.

Antacids should not be taken at the same time as vitamin C supplements because the alkaline compound neutralizes the ascorbic acid.

Megadoses of vitamin C taken during pregnancy may cause the newborn to require larger than average amounts of ascorbic acid.

See Table 11.1 for a summary of water- and fat-soluble vitamins.

Minerals

Minerals are chemical elements occuring in nature and in body fluids. The correct balance of each is required for maintenance of health. Minerals dissolved in the body fluids are called *electrolytes* because they carry positive or negative electrical charges required for body activities, such as conduction of nerve impulses, beating of the heart, skeletal muscle contraction, and absorption of nutrients from the gastrointestinal tract.

TABLE 11.1. SUMMARY OF WATER- AND FAT-SOLUBLE VITAMINS

Name	Food Sources	Functions	Deficiency/Toxicity

Vitamin A (retinol)	Animal
	    Liver
	    Whole milk
	    Butter
	    Cream
	    Cod liver oil
	Plants
	    Dark green leafy vegetables
	    Deep yellow or orange fruit
	    Fortified margarine
		Dim light vision
		Maintenance of mucous membranes
		Growth and development of bones
			Deficiency
			    Night blindness
			    Xerophthalmia
			    Respiratory infections
			    Bone growth ceases
			Toxicity
			    Cessation of menstruation
			    Joint pain
			    Stunted growth
			    Enlargement of liver

Vitamin D (cholecalciferol)	Animal
	    Eggs
	    Liver
	    Fortified milk
	Plants
	    None
		Bone growth	Deficiency
			    Rickets
			    Osteomalacia
			    Poorly developed teeth
			    Muscle spasms
			Toxicity
			    Kidney stones
			    Calcification of soft tissues

Vitamin E (alpha-tocopherol)	Animal
	    None
	Plant
	    Margarines
	    Salad dressing
		Antioxidant	Deficiency
			    Destruction of RBCs
			Toxicity
			    Hypertension

Vitamin K	Animal
	    Egg yolk
	    Liver
	    Milk
	Plant
	    Green leafy vegetables
	    Cabbage
		Blood clotting	Deficiency
			    Prolonged blood clotting
			Toxicity
			    Hemolytic anemia
			    Jaundice

Thiamin (Vitamin B_1)	Animal
	    Pork, beef
	    Liver
	    Eggs
	    Fish
	    Pork
	    Beef
	Plants
	    Whole and enriched grains
	    Legumes
		Coenzyme in oxidation of glucose	Deficiency
			    Gastrointestinal tract, nervous, and cardiovascular system problems
			Toxicity
			    None

Riboflavin (Vitamin B_2)	Animal
	    Milk
	Plants
	    Green vegetables
	    Cereals
	    Enriched bread
		Aids release of energy from food	Deficiency
			    Cheilosis
			    Glossitis
			    Photophobia
			Toxicity
			    None

Pyridoxine (Vitamin B_6)	Animal
	    Pork
	    Milk
	    Eggs
	Plants
	    Whole grain cereals
	    Legumes
		Synthesis of nonessential amino acids
		Conversion of tryptophan to niacin
		Antibody production
			Deficiency
			    Cheilosis
			    Glossitis
			Toxicity
			    Liver disease

Vitamin B_{12}	Animal
	    Seafood
	    Meat
	    Eggs
	    Milk
	Plants
	    None
		Synthesis of RBCs
		Maintenance of myelin sheaths
			Deficiency
			    Degeneration of myelin sheaths
			    Pernicious anemia
			Toxicity
			    None

TABLE 11.1 (Continued)

Name	Food Sources	Functions	Deficiency/Toxicity
Niacin (nicotinic acid)	Animal Milk Eggs Fish Poultry	Transfers hydrogen atoms for synthesis of ATP	Deficiency Pellagra Toxicity Vasodilation of blood vessels
Folacin	Animal None Plants Spinach Asparagus Broccoli Kidney beans	Synthesis of RBCs	Deficiency Glossitis Macrocytic anemia Toxicity None
Biotin	Animal Milk Liver Plants Legumes Mushrooms	Coenzyme in carbohydrate and amino acid metabolism Niacin synthesis from tryptophan	Deficiency None Toxicity None
Pantothenic acid	Animal Eggs Liver Salmon Yeast Plants Mushrooms Cauliflower Peanuts	Metabolism of carbohydrates, lipids, and proteins Synthesis of acetylcholine	Deficiency None Toxicity None
Vitamin C (ascorbic acid)	Fruits All citrus Plants Broccoli Tomatoes Brussel sprouts Potatoes	Prevention of scurvy Formation of collagen Healing of wounds Release of stress hormones Absorption of iron	Deficiency Scurvy Muscle cramps Ulcerated gums Toxicity Raise uric acid level Hemolytic anemia Kidney stones Rebound scurvy

Necessary for homeostasis (body balance), the correct ratio of fluids to electrolytes must be maintained for normal functioning of the body. Fluids and minerals are excreted daily and must be replaced with fluid and food intake.

The principal minerals in the body and their chemical symbols are sodium (Na), chloride (Cl), potassium (K), calcium (Ca), and iron (Fe).

SODIUM AND CHLORIDE

Sodium and chloride are the principal minerals in the intracellular body fluids. Blood contains approximately 0.9% sodium chloride.

Deficiencies of sodium and chloride are associated with:

Excessive fluid loss: bleeding, diarrhea, vomiting, or excessive perspiration
Insufficient oral intake

Treatment consists of intravenous therapy with sodium chloride (NaCl) according to needs:

Normal saline solution (0.9% sodium chloride)
Half-normal saline solution (0.45% sodium chloride)
Quarter-normal saline solution (0.2% sodium chloride)

Sometimes other minerals are required and are also added to the intravenous fluids.

POTASSIUM

Potassium is another of the principal minerals in the body fluids. Natural sources of potassium include citrus, bananas, tomatoes, potato skin, cantaloupe, and lima beans.

Necessary for:

Acid-base and fluid balance
Normal muscular irritability

Deficiencies are associated with:

Insufficient oral intake due to surgery, anorexia, or weight-reduction diets
Diarrhea or vomiting
Diabetic ketoacidosis
Diaphoresis (excessive perspiration)
Diuretic use, especially thiazides
Digitalis intoxication
Long-term use of corticosteroids

Signs of deficiency include:

Muscular weakness
Cardiac arrhythmias
Lethargy and fatigue

Treatment consists of:

IV KCl given postoperatively or with severe dehydration
One of the numerous oral products available, usually in effervescent tablet or powder form to be dissolved in water or juice and taken after meals (e.g., K-Lyte 50–100 mEq qd or Slow-K 40 mEq qd) or tablets to be swallowed (e.g., K-tabs of Micro K)

Side effects can include:

Nausea, vomiting, or diarrhea
GI bleeding

PATIENT EDUCATION

Patients should be instructed regarding:

Natural sources of potassium-rich foods

Conditions requiring potassium supplements

Directions for taking potassium supplements with or after meals to avoid GI distress

The importance of *dissolving* the tablet in solution *completely* before taking it and *never* holding the tablet in the mouth or swallowing the tablet whole

Notifying a doctor immediately of any side effects

CALCIUM

Calcium is a mineral component of bones and teeth. Natural sources include milk and dairy products (RDA, 1,000–1,200 mg/day).

Necessary for:

Strong bones and teeth
Normal muscle contraction
Nerve conduction
Blood coagulation

Deficiencies (supplements required) are associated with:

Pregnancy and lactation
Postmenopausal women (or those with estrogen deficiency)
Hypoparathyroidism
Long-term use of corticosteroids

Signs of deficiency may include:

Osteoporosis, including frequent fractures, especially in the elderly
Muscle pathology, including cardiac myopathy or tetany and leg cramps
Increased clotting time

Treatment consists of:

Calcium chloride, 0.5–1 g IV for cardiac arrest
Calcium gluconate, calcium carbonate, or calcium lactate, 1,000 to 1,200 mg daily for deficiency

Interactions may occur with:

Digitalis, resulting in potentiation (may cause arrhythmias)
Tetracycline, resulting in antagonism (inactivates the antibiotic)

> **PATIENT EDUCATION**
>
> Patients should be instructed regarding:
>
> Diet, foods that include dairy products
>
> Necessity for calcium supplements, especially for women, now recommended even before menopause
>
> Not taking calcium products at the same time as any other medication because, like other antacids, they have a neutralizing effect and inactivate many other medications

IRON

Iron is a mineral found in meat (especially liver), egg yolk, beans, spinach, and enriched cereals.

Necessary for hemoglobin formation.

Deficiencies (supplements recommended) are associated with:

Hemorrhage and excessive menstrual flow
Internal bleeding, ulcers, and GI tumors
Pregnancy
Infancy

Signs of deficiency may include:

Paleness of the skin and/or mucous membranes
Lethargy and weakness
Vertigo
Air hunger

Treatment of anemia due to iron deficiency consists of administration of iron preparations:

Oral iron products. Ferrous sulfate (Feosol, Fer-in-sol, and others); adults, 50–100 mg tid after meals (not with milk, coffee, or tea) infants and children, 4–6 mg/kg tid in juice or with meals (not with milk).

Injectable iron. Iron dextran (Imferon) 50–250 mg *deep* IM by the *Z-track method only*. Extreme caution is urged to prevent solution contacting the subcutaneous tissue because of its irritating effect. A fresh 2-inch needle is recommended at the time of administration. Iron dextran also can be given IV *slowly* after testing for sensitivity with a small trial dose.

Side effects of taking iron preparations can include:

Black stools
Nausea and vomiting (GI effects can be minimized by taking iron after or with meals)

Constipation or diarrhea
Anaphylactic reactions or phlebitis with IV administration of iron dextran

Interactions may occur with:

Vitamin C, taken at same time, which enhances iron absorption
Coffee or tea taken within 2 hours of iron, which reduces iron absorption by as much as 50%
Tetracycline, absorption of which is inhibited by oral iron preparations when taken within 2 hours
Antacids, which decrease iron absorption (should not be given at same time)

Symptoms of overdose include:

Lethargy
Shock
Vomiting and diarrhea
Erosion of GI tract

PATIENT EDUCATION

Patients should be instructed regarding:

Avoidance of self-medication without established need (blood test) and without medical supervision to determine why hemoglobin is low. Taking iron when not prescribed could mask the symptoms of internal bleeding or GI malignancy.
Black stools to be expected.
Taking iron at meals to minimize GI distress.
Interactions (i.e., avoidance of coffee, tea, or antacids at same time).
Caution with flavored children's tablets (overdosage can be dangerous).

ZINC

Zinc is an essential element in metabolism. It is usually found in adequate amounts in a well-balanced diet.

Necessary for wound healing.

Deficiencies (supplements recommended) are associated with:

Inadequate diet
Chronic, nonhealing wounds
Major surgery or trauma

Treatment consists of 200–220 mg tablets or capsules administered with meals tid to minimize gastric distress.

Many combinations of various vitamins and minerals are available in over-the-counter products with various strengths and forms.

PATIENT EDUCATION

Patients should be instructed regarding:

    Well-balanced diets and sources of vitamins and minerals
    Food preparation to avoid loss of vitamins
    Information regarding signs of·deficiency and overdose
    Caution in taking supplements without established need or without medical supervision, especially megadoses, fat-soluble vitamins, and iron
    Proper administration to minimize side effects

See Table 11.2 for a summary of the major minerals.

TABLE 11.2. SUMMARY OF MAJOR MINERALS

Name	Food Sources	Functions	Deficiency/Toxicity

Calcium (Ca)	Milk exchanges
	  Milk, cheese
	Meat exchanges
	  Sardines
	  Salmon
	Vegetable exchanges
	  Green vegetables
		Development of bones and teeth
		Permeability of cell membranes
		Transmission of nerve impulses
		Blood clotting
			Deficiency
			  Osteoporosis
			  Osteomalacia
			  Rickets

Phosphorus (P)	Milk exchanges
	  Milk, cheese
	Meat exchanges
	  Lean meat
		Development of bones and teeth
		Transfer of energy
		Component of phospholipids
		Buffer system
			(Same as calcium)

Potassium (K)	Fruit exchanges
	  Oranges, bananas
	  Dried fruits
		Contraction of muscles
		Maintaining water balance
		Transmission of nerve impulses
		Carbohydrate and protein
		  metabolism
			Deficiency
			  Hypokalemia
			Toxicity
			  Hyperkalemia

Sodium (Na)	Table salt
	Meat exchanges
	  Beef, eggs
	Milk exchanges
	  Milk, cheese
		Maintaining fluid balance in
		  blood
		Transmission of nerve impulses
			Toxicity
			  Increase in blood
			  pressure

Chlorine (Cl)	Table salt
	Meat exchanges
		Gastric acidity
		Regulation of osmotic pressure
		Activation of salivary amylase
			Deficiency
			  Imbalance in gastric
			  acidity
			  Imbalance in blood pH

Magnesium (Mg)	Vegetable exchanges
	  Green vegetables
	Bread exchanges
	  Whole grains
		Synthesis of ATP
		Transmission of nerve impulses
		Activator of metabolic enzymes
		Relaxation of skeletal muscles	

Sulfur (S)	Meat exchanges
	  Eggs, poultry, fish
		Maintaining protein structure
		Formation of high-energy
		  compounds	

WORKSHEET 1 FOR CHAPTER 11

Fat-Soluble Vitamins

List the fat-soluble vitamins and complete all columns.

VITAMIN	SOURCES	CAUSE OF DEFICIENCIES	SIGNS OF DEFICIENCIES	SYMPTOMS OF OVERDOSE	INTERACTIONS AND CAUTIONS

WORKSHEET 2 FOR CHAPTER 11

Water-Soluble Vitamins

List water-soluble vitamin names and complete all columns.

VITAMIN AND NAME	SOURCES	CAUSE OF DEFICIENCIES	SIGNS OF DEFICIENCIES	SYMPTOMS OF OVERDOSE	INTERACTIONS AND CAUTIONS
B_1					
B_2					
B_6					
B_{12}					
Folic acid					
Niacin					

WORKSHEET 3 FOR CHAPTER 11

Vitamins and Minerals

List the vitamin names and mineral symbols, and complete all columns.

VITAMIN WITH NAME MINERALS WITH SYMBOL	SOURCES	CAUSE OF DEFICIENCIES	SIGNS OF DEFICIENCIES	SYMPTOMS OF OVERDOSE	INTERACTIONS AND CAUTIONS
C					
Potassium					
Calcium					
Iron					

12

Skin Medications

OBJECTIVES

Upon completion of this chapter, the student will be able to:

1. Define antipruritic, emollient, demulcent, keratolytic, antiseptic, disinfectant, bactericidal, and bacteriostatic.
2. Describe application procedures for various skin preparations.
3. Identify side effects of the six major categories of skin preparations and contraindications when appropriate.
4. Compare and contrast scabicides and pediculicides.
5. Explain the factors that influence the absorption of skin medications.
6. Classify drugs according to their action: antipruritic, emollient, keratolytic, antifungal, or anti-infective.
7. Describe important patient education for all skin medications in this chapter.

The skin is the largest organ of the body. Since such a great area is involved, many conditions can affect the skin, causing annoyance and discomfort. Skin ailments can range from minor ones, such as pruritis (itching), to major ones, such as severe burns. Treatment is usually topical or local (applied to the affected area), but skin conditions are sometimes treated internally with oral medications or injections for their systemic effects.

This chapter explains *topical* medications only. Medications given parenterally or orally to relieve inflammation or itching, such as corticosteroids and antihistamines, are discussed in other chapters.

Topical skin preparations can be classified according to action in six principal categories:

1. Antipruritics relieve itching.
2. Emollients and demulcents soothe irritation.
3. Keratolytic agents loosen epithelial scales.
4. Scabicides and pediculicides treat scabies or lice.
5. Antifungals control fungus conditions.
6. Local anti-infectives prevent and treat infection.

Factors that influence the rate of absorption of medication include condition and location of the skin, heat, and moisture. If the skin is thick and callused, absorption will be slower. If the skin is moist, macerated (raw), or warm, absorption will be more rapid. Sometimes the physician will order that the skin be premoistened or plastic wrap be applied over the ointment to aid absorption; in other cases, the skin must be left exposed to the air to slow absorption and reduce systemic effects. At times, the length of time for the medication to remain on the skin is very important. Complete understanding of appropriate directions for each topical medication is vital *before administration*.

Antipruritics

Antipruritics relieve itching by use of products singly or in combination containing:

Local anesthetics (e.g., the "-caines," such as benzocaine)
Drying agents
Anti-inflammatory agents (e.g., corticosteroids) applied locally or given PO for systemic effect
Antihistamines administered PO for systemic effect

They are used to relieve discomfort from dermatitis (rashes) associated with allergic reactions, poison ivy, hives, and insect bites.

Side effects can include:

Skin irritation
Stinging and a burning sensation
Allergic reactions (especially with the "-caines")

Contraindications include:

For prolonged use (especially corticosteroids)
The "-caines" for allergic persons

PATIENT EDUCATION

Patients should be instructed to:

Use caution if they have allergies.
Avoid contact with eyes or mucous membranes.
Avoid covering with dressings unless directed by physician.
Avoid prolonged use (not longer than 1 week).
Discontinue if condition worsens or irritation develops.
Trim children's fingernails to reduce possibility of infection.

Emollients and Demulcents

Emollients and demulcents are used topically to protect or soothe minor dermatological conditions, such as diaper rash, abrasions, and minor burns.

Keratolytics

Keratolytic agents are used to control conditions of abnormal scaling of the skin, such as dandruff, seborrhea, and psoriasis, or to promote peeling of the skin in conditions such as acne, hard corns, calluses, and warts.

Side effects can include:

Severe skin irritation
Irritation to eyes or mucous membranes
Photosensitivity
Systemic effects in allergic individuals (e.g., headache and GI symptoms)
Increased susceptibility to skin cancer (only with prolonged use for many years)

Contraindications include:

Pregnancy and lactation
Small children
For prolonged periods of time

PATIENT EDUCATION

Patients should be instructed to:

Avoid contact with eyes and mucous membranes.
Avoid prolonged use.
Discontinue and seek medical aid if irritation occurs.
Avoid contact with surrounding tissues when applied as a caustic to corns or calluses.

See Table 12.1 for a summary of antipruritics, emollients, and keratolytics.

TABLE 12.1. TOPICAL MEDICATIONS FOR THE SKIN: ANTIPRURITICS, EMOLLIENTS, DEMULCENTS, AND KERATOLYTICS

Generic Name	Trade Name	Available	Comments
Antipruritics			
benzocaine	Americaine	Ointment, spray	
calamine	Caladryl (with Benadryl)	Lotion	Drying
		Lotion, ointment	Antihistamine
corticosteroid	Cortaid, Topicort, many others	Ointment, cream	Reduced resistance to infection
Emollients and Demulcents			
vitamins A and D	A & D	Ointment	
	Desitin (with zinc oxide)	Ointment	
Keratolytics			
coal tar	Zetar, Tegrin, Neutrogena	Shampoo, lotion	
podophyllum	Podophyllin	Sol	For anogenital warts; systemic toxicity possible
salicylic acid	Many combinations with other keratolytics	Ointment, sol, shampoo	For dandruff, psoriasis, warts, corns, calluses
sulfur	Cuticura, Clearasil	Cream, gel, lotion, shampoo	For acne, dandruff; for scabies in infants

Note: This table lists only typical medications and does not include all of those on the market.

Scabicides and Pediculicides

Scabies is caused by an itch mite that burrows under the skin. It is easily transmitted from one person to another by direct contact or through contact with contaminated clothing or bed linens. Effective treatment includes laundering in hot water or dry cleaning all clothing and bedding.

Scabicides (benzyl benzoate or lindane) must be applied *according to directions* on the package insert, left in place the required period of time, and then rinsed thoroughly. The most effective pediculicide is considered to be lindane (Kwell).

Side effects, rare when applied *topically according to directions,* may include:

Slight local irritation
Dermatitis with frequent application

However, with excessive or prolonged use or with oral ingestion, CNS symptoms, hepatic, or renal toxicity may occur.

Contraindications include:

- Acutely inflamed, raw, or weeping surfaces.
- Since lindane (Kwell) can be absorbed systemically following topical application, it should be avoided during pregnancy, lactation or with infants and small children.

However, benzyl benzoate is a safe alternative under these conditions.

PATIENT EDUCATION

Patients should be instructed to:

Thoroughly launder clothing and bedding.
Use caution to prevent accidental oral ingestion.
Use caution with infants who might suck thumbs.

Antifungals

Antifungals are useful in the treatment of monilial infections (candidiasis), such as thrush, diaper rash, vaginitis; and ringworm, such as athlete's foot and jock itch.

Effective treatment includes topical administration according to directions on the package insert and good hygiene practices, including washing, drying, and exposure to air when possible.

Side effects, although rare, may include:

Contact dermatitis
Itching, burning, and irritation

Contraindication or caution (under medical supervision only) applies to the use of vaginal preparations during pregnancy.

PATIENT EDUCATION

Patients should be instructed to:

Carefully wash and *dry* affected areas.
Expose to air whenever possible.
Avoid tight undergarments, pantyhose, and wet bathing suits with genital fungus.
Use open sandals instead of sneakers with athlete's foot.
Follow application instructions carefully.
Remove any stains with soap and warm water.
Continue prescribed vaginal treatment even during menstruation or if symptomatic relief occurs until entire regime is completed.
Consult doctor before vaginal preparations are used during pregnancy.

Local Anti-infectives

ANTISEPTICS

Antiseptics are substances that inhibit the growth of bacteria (bacteriostatic). The term is used most frequently to describe chemicals applied to body tissues, especially the skin. *Disinfectants* are included in this category, but chemicals that kill bacteria (bactericidal) are frequently too strong to be applied to body tissues and are *usually* applied to inanimate objects, such as furniture, floors, and instruments. Sometimes a chemical can be used as an antiseptic on skin and also as a disinfectant on inanimate objects by increasing the strength.

The two major antiseptics in use today are hexachlorophene and iodine, used for surgical scrubs and as bacteriostatic skin cleansers. Some iodine preparations are also bactericidal and are used in the treatment of superficial skin wounds and to disinfect the skin preoperatively.

Side effects of hexachlorophene can be serious and *rinsing thoroughly* after its use is vital to prevent:

Dermatitis and reddness
Photosensitivity
Systemic effects (e.g., CNS irritability, seizures, and death)

Side effects of iodine can include:

Skin irritation or burns
Allergic reactions

Contraindications or extreme cautions for hexachlorophene include:

Not for frequent use for total body bathing
Not for routine use for infants, especially with premature or low-birth-weight infants (rinse well)

Never on burned, open skin or mucous membranes
Not for use with occlusive dressings

Iodine cautions include:

Not for those allergic to iodine
Not covering with tight bandage

PATIENT EDUCATION

Patients should be instructed to:

Rinse hexachlorophene *thoroughly*.
Avoid hexachlorophene for total body bathing, especially with small infants.
Avoid use of hexachlorophene on open skin lesions, mucous membranes, and genital areas.
Take care to avoid hexachlorophene or iodine in the eyes; flush thoroughly.
Avoid tight dressings over both medications.
Use caution with iodine in anyone with allergies.
Keep tincture of iodine bottles closed tightly to prevent evaporation of alcohol, leading to increase in strength and possible iodine burns.

BURN MEDICATIONS

Burn treatments include application of medications to prevent or treat infections. The two most commonly used agents for this purpose are nitrofurazone (Furacin) and silver sulfadiazine (Silvadene).

Side effects can include:

Pain, burning, and itching
Allergic reactions

Contraindications or extreme caution applies to patients with:

Impaired kidney or liver function (cumulative effects)
History of allergy, especially to sulfa drugs
Newborns

PATIENT EDUCATION

Patients should be instructed to:

Use aseptic technique to prevent infection.
Watch for allergic reactions.
Keep careful intake and output record.

TABLE 12.2. TOPICAL MEDICATIONS FOR THE SKIN: SCABICIDES, PEDICULICIDES, ANTIFUNGALS, ANTISEPTICS, AND BURN MEDICATIONS

Generic Name	Trade Name	Available	Comments
Scabicides and Pediculicides			
benzyl benzoate		Lotion	Apply two coats to remain 24 h
lindane	Kwell	Cream, lotion, shampoo	Treat all hairy areas
Antifungals[a]			
amphotericin B	Fungizone	Cream, lotion, ointment	May stain skin, nails, or clothes
nystatin	Mycostatin	Oral suspension, cream, lotion, ointment vaginal tab	
tolnaftate	Tinactin	Aerosol spray cream, powder, sol	Avoid inhaling spray or powder
zinc undecylenate	Cruex, Desenex	Aerosol spray, powder ointment, cream	Spray or powder
Topical Anti-infectives and Antiseptics			
hexachlorophene	Phisohex, Septisol	Sol, liquid soap	Bacteriostatic skin cleanser, surgical scrub; rinse thoroughly
povidone-iodine	Betadine, Efodine	Aq sol, tinct, liquid scrub	Bactericidal, antiseptic, surgical scrub; watch for allergies
Burn Medications			
nitrofurazone	Furacin	Cream, ointment sol	Watch for allergies
silver sulfadiazine	Silvadene	Cream	Watch for allergies

[a]Oral preparations are discussed in Chapter 13.

See Table 12.2 for a summary of scabicides, pediculicides, antifungals, antiseptics, and burn medications.

Cautions for Topical Medications

Skin medications by prescription or over-the-counter are too numerous to mention. Many patients use products without adequate instruction in administration, side effects, or precautions. The health worker has a responsibility to advise patients whenever possible to use great caution with self-medication to avoid ineffective or dangerous treatment. Both the health worker and the layperson should read instructions completely before administration of any medication.

PATIENT EDUCATION

Patients using topical medications should be instructed regarding:

Never taking by mouth
Keeping out of reach of children
Being sure labels are not obscured and are read completely
Discontinuing at once with any side effects and seeking medical advice
Not taking beyond time limit listed on medication container
If allergies are known, avoiding self-medication without medical advice

WORKSHEET FOR CHAPTER 12

Drugs for the Skin

List the drugs according to category and complete all columns. Learn generic or trade names as specified by instructor.

CLASSIFICATIONS AND DRUGS	PURPOSE	SIDE EFFECTS	CONTRAINDICATIONS OR CAUTIONS	PATIENT EDUCATION
Antipruritics				
1.				
2.				
3.				
Emollients and Demulcents				
1.				
Kerolytics				
1.				
2.				
3.				
4.				
Scabicides and Pediculicides				
1.				
2.				

CLASSIFICATIONS AND DRUGS	PURPOSE	SIDE EFFECTS	CONTRAINDICATIONS OR CAUTIONS	PATIENT EDUCATION
Antifungals 1. 2. 3. 4.				
Antiseptics 1. 2.				
Burn Medications 1. 2.				

13

Anti-infective Drugs

OBJECTIVES

Upon completion of this chapter, the student will be able to:

1. Define C & S, broad-spectrum, resistance, hypersensitivity, anaphylaxis, direct and indirect toxicity, and superinfection.
2. Identify side effects, contraindications, and interactions common to each category of anti-infectives listed in Tables 13.1, 13.2, and 13.3.
3. Explain the unique features of patient education appropriate for each category of anti-infectives.
4. Describe general instructions that should be given to every patient undergoing anti-infective therapy.

Treatment of infection with medication is complicated by the great variety of these medications available and the differing modes of action of the various drugs (e.g., bacteriostatic versus bactericidal). The first step in treatment is identification of the causative organism and the specific medication to which it is sensitive. *Culture and sensitivity tests (C & S)* will be ordered, based on symptoms, (e.g., wound, throat, urine, or blood). It is imperative to obtain the appropriate specimen before administering medication. Results of C & S will not be available for 24–48 h. In the meantime, the physician will frequently order a *broad-spectrum* antibiotic, one that is effective against a large variety of organisms.

Sometimes organisms build up *resistance* to drugs that have been used too frequently, and then the drugs are no longer effective. This explains why antibiotics are not used for the common cold, which is usually caused by a virus rather than a bacteria anyway. Organisms can also become resistant if infections have been treated incompletely, as when the medication is discontinued before the required number of days to be fully effective.

Adverse reactions to anti-infectives are divided into three categories:

1. *Allergic hypersensitivity.* Overresponse of the body to a specific substance. A *mild* reaction with only rash, urticaria (hives), or mild fever, is usually treated with corticosteroids or antihistamines, and the medication is *discontinued*. Sometimes severe reactions occur with the first administration of a specific medication (e.g., penicillin), or they may follow a mild reaction. *Severe* reactions may be manifested as *anaphylaxis*, a sudden onset of dyspnea, chest constriction, shock, and collapse. Unless treated promptly with epinephrine, corticosteroids, and CPR, death may result.

2. *Direct toxicity.* Results in tissue damage, such as ototoxicity (hearing difficulties or dizziness), nephrotoxicity (kidney problems), hepatotoxity (liver damage), or blood dyscracias (abnormalities in blood components). Sometimes the damage is permanent, or it may be reversible when the medication is discontinued. The health worker's responsibility involves assessment of physical condition and laboratory reports, and *discontinuance* of medication at the first sign of toxicity.

3. *Indirect toxicity, or superinfection.* Manifested as a new infection with different resistant bacteria or fungi as a result of killing the normal flora in the intestines or mucous membranes. Symptoms of superinfections can include diarrhea, vaginitis, stomatitis, or glossitis. Treatment consists of antifungal medications and including buttermilk or yogurt in the diet to restore normal intestinal flora. With the other two types of adverse reactions, the medication is discontinued. With superinfections, the medication is *continued*, the symptoms are treated, and sometimes the dosage is adjusted.

It would be impractical to list all the anti-infective agents on the market. Therefore, only a few examples of the most frequently used drugs are listed in each category. The antibiotics are divided into six categories: aminoglycosides, cephalosporins, chloramphenicol, erythromycins, penicillins, and tetracyclines. In addition, antifungals, antituberculosis agents, antivirals, sulfonamides, and urinary anti-infectives are also listed. We have omitted the amebicides, anthelmintics, and antimalarial drugs but urge those in the public health or pediatric fields to investigate these drugs as appropriate to their practice.

Aminoglycosides

Aminoglycosides are used to treat many infections caused by gram-negative bacteria (e.g., *Pseudomonas* and *Salmonella*) as well as many gram-positive bacteria, (e.g., *Staphylococcus aureus*). Aminoglycosides are used in the *short-term* treatment of many serious infections (e.g., septicemia) *only* when other less toxic anti-infectives are ineffective or contraindicated. Examples of aminoglycosides include gentamycin and tobramycin.

Serious side effects, especially in the elderly or those with renal or hearing impairment, can include:

Nephrotoxicity, including pathologic kidney condition
Ototoxicity, both auditory (hearing loss) and vestibular (vertigo)
Neuromuscular blocking, including respiratory paralysis
CNS symptoms, including headache, tremor, lethargy, rash, and urticaria

Contraindications or extreme caution applies to patients with:

Tinnitus, vertigo, and high-frequency hearing loss
Reduced renal function
Dehydration
Pregnancy

Interactions may occur with:

Other ototoxic drugs (e.g., amphotericin B, cephalosporins, and polymixin B)
General anesthetics or neuromuscular blocking agents (e.g., succinylcholine or curare), which can cause respiratory paralysis
Diuretics such as furosemide (Lasix)

PATIENT EDUCATION

Patients should be instructed regarding:

Extreme importance of close medical supervision during therapy
Careful observation of intake and urinary output
Prompt reporting of any side effects, especially kidney or hearing problems

---

Cephalosporins

Cephalosporins are broad-spectrum antibiotics used to treat serious infections of respiratory tract, skin, urinary tract, and bones and joints; endocarditis; some septicemias; some meningitis; and some pelvic inflammatory disease (PID). They are also used prophylactically, especially in high-risk patients, for many types of surgery. Less toxic than the aminoglycosides, they are effective against many of the same organisms as penicillin. Examples include cephalexin and cefotaxime.

Side effects can include:

Hypersensitivity, including rash, edema, or anaphylaxis (especially in those allergic to penicillin)
Blood dyscracias (e.g., increased bleeding time)
Renal toxicity, especially in older patients
Mild hepatic dysfunction
Nausea, vomiting, and diarrhea
Phlebitis with IV administration and pain at site of IM injection
False-positive Clinitest results in diabetics

Contraindications or extreme caution applies to:

Known allergies, especially to penicillin (3%–6% cross-sensitivity)
Prolonged use possibly leading to superinfections
Pregnancy

Interactions can include:

Increased effectiveness with probenecid
Adverse reactions (flushing or shock) with alcohol ingestion

PATIENT EDUCATION

Patients should be instructed regarding:

Possible allergic reactions
Avoidance of alcohol
Reporting any side effects to physician
Including buttermilk or yogurt in diet to restore normal intestinal flora
Taking without regard to meals but with food if stomach upset occurs
Attention to signs of abnormal bleeding (checking stools and urine for blood)

Chloramphenicol

Chloramphenicol (Chloromycetin) is potentially very toxic and therefore is used only to treat serious infections caused by susceptible organisms when less toxic drugs are ineffective. It is used for typhoid fever, meningitis (*Hemophilus influenzae*), rickettsial infections (e.g., Rocky Mountain spotted fever), or bacteremia when other antibiotics have proven ineffective.

Serious side effects can include:

Bone marrow depression, leading to bleeding and infections
Aplastic anemia, which can be fatal
Circulatory collapse, which can lead to death
Visual disturbances
Neuritis, headache, and confusion

Interactions can occur with:

Potentiation of dicumarol, phenytoin, and tolbutamide
Antagonistic response to vitamin B_{12}, folic acid, or iron preparations

---

PATIENT EDUCATION

Patients should be instructed regarding the very serious potential side effects of chloramphenicol and given explanations regarding its use when absolutely necessary under close medical supervision.

Erythromycins

Erythromycins are used in many infections of the respiratory tract and for skin conditions such as acne or for some sexually transmitted infections when the patient is allergic to penicillin. Erythromycins are considered among the least toxic antibiotics and are therefore preferred for treating susceptible organisms under conditions in which more toxic antibiotics might be dangerous (e.g., in patients with renal disease, pregnant patients, or small infants).

Side effects of a serious nature are rare, and mild side effects, usually dose-related, can include:

Anorexia, nausea, vomiting, diarrhea, and cramps
Urticaria and rash
Superinfections

Contraindications or caution applies to patients with:

Liver dysfunction
Alcoholism

PATIENT EDUCATION

Patients should be instructed regarding:

Common GI side effects to be expected

Importance of reporting side effects for possible dosage adjustment or prescription of medication for symptomatic relief

Taking medication with full glass of water on empty stomach unless stomach upset (some forms can be taken without regard to meals)

Including yogurt or buttermilk in diet to help regulate intestinal flora and reduce incidence of diarrhea

---

Penicillins

Penicillins are antibiotics used to treat many streptococcal and some staphylococcal and meningococcal infections, including respiratory and intestinal infections. Penicillin is the drug of choice for treatment of gonorrhrea and syphilis, and is also used prophylactically to prevent recurrences of rheumatic fever. Some semisynthetic penicillins have a wider spectrum of activity and are called extended-spectrum penicillins.

Serious side effects of penicillins can include:

Hypersensitivity reactions ranging from rash to fatal anaphylaxis
Superinfections (especially with oral ampicillin)
Nausea, vomiting, and diarrhea
Blood dyscracias, which are reversible with discontinuance of drug
Fever

Contraindications or extreme caution applies to patients with:

History of allergy, especially to any drugs (anaphylaxis has been reported with parenteral, oral, or intradermal skin testing)

Treatment for severe reactions includes discontinuance of the drug, immediate administration of appropriate medications (e.g., epinephrine and corticosteroids), and maintenance of a patent airway.

Interactions include:

Potentiation of penicillin with probenecid (Benemid) and with anti-inflammatory drugs such as phenylbutazone, indomethacin, and the salicylates given concomitantly (at the same time)

Antagonistic effect (delayed absorption) of oral penicillins when given with antacids or with food

TABLE 13.1. ANTI-INFECTIVE AGENTS: AMINOGLYCOSIDES, CEPHALOSPORINS, CHLORAMPHENICOL, ERYTHROMYCINS, AND PENICILLINS

Generic Name	Trade Name	Average Dosage
Aminoglycosides		
gentamycin	Garamycin	IM, IV 1 mg/kg body weight q8h
neomycin	Mycifradin	Oral sol, tab, IV 40–88 mg qd in divided doses
tobramycin	Nebcin	IM, IV 1 mg/kg body weight q8h
Cephalosporins		
cephalexin	Keflex	Cap, liquid, tab 250 mg q6h
cephamandole	Mandol	IV, deep IM 500 mg–1 g q4–8h
cefotaxime	Claforin	IV, deep IM 1 g q6–8h
Chloramphenicol		
chloramphenicol	Chloromycetin	Oral 50 mg/kg body weight qd IV 50 mg/kg body weight qd in divided doses q6h
Erythromycins		
	E-Mycin, Ilosone	Tab, cap 250–500 mg q6h
	EES	Tab, suspension 400 mg q6h
	Erythrocin, Ilotysin	IV dosage determined by condition treated
Penicillins		
	Amoxicillin, Ampicillin	Cap, tab, suspension 250–500 mg q6–8h
carbenicillin	Geopen	IV (continuous or div. doses) 400–500 mg/kg body weight qd
ticarcillin	Ticar	IV div. doses 200–300 mg/kg body weight qd
penicillin G procaine	Bicillin, Crystacillin, Wycillin	Deep IM 600,000–1.2 million U
penicillin VK	V-Cillin K, Pen-Vee K	Tab 250–500 mg q6h

Note: Average doses only are listed. In severe infections, higher doses may be indicated. Many other anti-infectives are available. Only a few are represented here.

> **PATIENT EDUCATION**
>
> Patients should be instructed regarding:
>
> Discontinuance of medication and *immediate* reporting of any hypersensitivity reactions (e.g., rash, swelling, or difficulty breathing)
> Taking medication on time as prescribed on empty stomach with full glass of water
> Avoidance of antacids and alcohol

See Table 13.1 for a summary of the aminoglycosides, cephalosporins, chloramphenicol, erythromycins, and penicillins.

Tetracyclines

Tetracyclines are broad-spectrum antibiotics used for a variety of bacterial infections (e.g., rickettsial, or Rocky Mountain spotted fever), atypical pneumonia, some sexually transmitted infections, and some severe cases of inflammatory acne. However, some organisms are showing increasing resistance to the tetracyclines, and therefore they should be used only when other antibiotics are ineffective or contraindicated.

Side effects can include:

Nausea, vomiting, and diarrhea (frequently dose-related)
Superinfections such as vaginitis and stomatitis
Photosensitivity, with exaggerated sunburn
Discolored teeth in fetus or young children
Retarded bone growth in fetus or young children
Hepatic or renal toxicity (rare)
CNS symptoms (rare) such as vertigo and cerebral edema
Thrombophlebitis possible with IV therapy

Contraindications include:

Pregnancy, lactation and children under age 8
Patients exposed to direct sunlight
Caution in patients with liver or kidney disease

Interactions may occur with the following antagonists (which decrease absorption):

Antacids
Iron preparations
Calcium supplements
Magnesium laxatives

Antidiarrhea agents containing kaolin, pectin, or bismuth
Dairy products

PATIENT EDUCATION

Patients should be instructed regarding:

Avoiding exposure to sunlight
Avoiding this medication if pregnant or nursing or a child under 8 years of age
Administration preferable on empty stomach with full glass of water, unless there is gastric distress
Avoiding iron, calcium, magnesium, and antidiarrhea agents or dairy foods within 3 h of taking tetracyclines

---

Antifungals

Antifungal agents are used to treat specific susceptible fungi. The medications are quite different in action and purpose, and are treated separately.

AMPHOTERICIN B

Amphotericin B is used for the treatment of severe systemic, potentially fatal, infections caused by susceptible fungi. *Severe side effects* are expected, and therefore close medical supervision (hospitalization) is usually required so that measures are available to provide symptomatic relief (e.g., antipyretics, antihistamines, and antiemetics).

Side effects include several of the following:

Headache, chills, and fever
Malaise, muscle and joint pain, and weakness
Anorexia, nausea, vomiting, and cramps
Nephrotoxicity
Anemia

GRISEOFULVIN

Griseofulvin is used in the treatment of specific fungi causing *tinea* infections (e.g., ringworm or athlete's foot).

Side effects can include:

Headache
Thirst, nausea, vomiting, and diarrhea

Rash
Photosensitivity
Hepatic toxicity

Contraindications include:

Pregnancy
Liver dysfunction

Interactions may occur with:

Alcohol, causing flushing and tachycardia
Phenobarbital, which is antagonistic to griseofulvin action

NYSTATIN

Nystatin (Mycostatin) is used in the treatment of monilial (candidal) infections of the mucous membranes (intestines, vagina, and mouth). It is also used in the topical treatment of skin and mucous membranes.

Side effects are rare but may include nausea, vomiting, and diarrhea with high oral doses occasionally.

No *contraindications* or *interactions* exist.

PATIENT EDUCATION

Patients with fungal infections should be instructed regarding:

Keeping affected area clean and dry
Exposure to air whenever possible
Avoidance of plastic pants, pantyhose, girdles, and sneakers (depending on area affected)

Antituberculosis Agents

Antituberculosis agents are administered for two purposes: (1) to treat asymptomatic infection (no evidence of clinical disease), for instance, after exposure to active tuberculosis and/or significantly positive PPD skin test and; (2) for treatment of active clinical tuberculosis and to prevent relapse.

For asymptomatic tuberculosis, the *treatment* consists of daily administration of isoniazid (INH) alone for 12 months to prevent development of the disease. On the other hand, to treat clinical tuberculosis and to prevent relapse, administration of at least two antitubercular agents is required for *prolonged periods of time*, (9–24 months, depending on severity and prior treatment). Patient compliance with consistent treatment over the required period of time is absolutely necessary to prevent relapse.

Side effects of INH and rifampin are usually more pronounced in the first few weeks of therapy and can be treated symptomatically. Dosage regulations are sometimes required in cases of acute toxicity, but the medication must *not* be discontinued. Side effects can include:

Nausea, vomiting, and diarrhea
Dizziness, blurred vision, headache, and fatigue
Numbness, weakness of extremities
Hepatic toxicity
Ototoxicity and nephrotoxicity *only* with streptomycin, an aminoglycoside
Excretions colored red-orange with rifampin
Hypersensitivity reaction, with flulike symptoms (sometimes with rifampin)

Contraindications or caution applies to patients with:

Chronic liver disease or alcoholics, periodic laboratory tests required
Impaired renal function
Pregnancy and lactation

Interactions include:

Antagonism by oral hypoglycemics, corticosteroids, digitalis, anticoagulants, and estrogen (serum levels of these drugs are reduced when taking rifampin)
Potentiation by phenytoin (Dilantin); increased action (possible toxicity) when taken with Isoniazid.
Alcohol, which increases possibility of liver toxicity

PATIENT EDUCATION

Patients should be instructed regarding:

Taking prescribed medication for lengthy required period of time, even though asymptomatic
Reporting side effects for possible dosage adjustment or prescription of other palliative medications to relieve discomfort
Importance of frequent medical and laboratory checks
Red-orange color of urine, feces, sputum, sweat, and tears with use of rifampin
Interactions with other drugs, (e.g., birth control pills may be ineffective)
Avoidance of alcohol

See Table 13.2 for a summary of the tetracyclines, antifungals, and antituberculosis agents.

TABLE 13.2. ANTI-INFECTIVE AGENTS: TETRACYCLINES, ANTIFUNGALS, AND ANTITUBERCULOSIS AGENTS

Generic Name	Trade Name	Average Dosage	Comments
Tetracyclines			
tetracycline HCl	Achromycin	Cap, tab, suspension, IV 150–500 mg q6–8h	
doxycycline	Vibramycin	Cap, tab, suspension, IV 100–200 mg qd	
oxytetracycline	Terramycin	Cap, tab, suspension, IM, IV 1–2 g qd in divided doses	
Antifungals			
amphotericin B	Fungizone	IV dose depends on condition treated	Special IV cautions, protect from light
griseofulvin	Grisactin, Fulvicin	Cap, tab, suspension 250 mg–1 g qd	
nystatin	Mycostatin	Tab, suspension 500,000–1 million U tid	
Antituberculosis Agents			
isoniazid	INH	Tab 5–10 mg/kg body weight qid 1 dose	Preventive alone, as treatment with other medications
ethambutol	Myambutol	Tab 15 mg/kg body weight qid 1 dose	Always with other medications
rifampin	Rifadin	Deep IM 600 mg qid 1 dose	Always with other medications
streptomycin	Streptomycin		Always with other medications

Antivirals

Antiviral (acyclovir) is used predominantly in the treatment of herpes simplex and herpes zoster infections. Acyclovir does *not* cure or prevent further occurrence of blisterlike lesions. Topical application appears effective only with initial infections in relieving discomfort and shortening healing time of lesions. Parenteral treatment is most effective in initial treatment of herpes to relieve pain and to speed healing of lesions. Effectiveness of acyclovir in treatment of reoccurrences of lesions following initial infections is under investigation.

Side effects are not common, but can include:

Impaired renal function
Lethargy, tremors, and confusion
Rash, urticaria, and inflammation at injection site
Nausea, vomiting, and abdominal pain
Reversible blood dyscracias

Contraindications or *caution* applies to patients with:

Renal or hepatic disease
Dehydration
Neurologic abnormalities

PATIENT EDUCATION

Patients should be instructed regarding:

The fact that acyclovir is usually effective only with *initial* infection in relieving pain and shortening healing of lesions, but is *not* a cure and there will be recurrences of lesions

Applying ointment to the skin *carefully* with a finger cot, which is then discarded so as to prevent spread of the infection to other sites or other persons

Taking care to keep acyclovir *out of the eyes*

Sulfonamides

Sulfonamides are among the oldest anti-infectives. They are in limited use today because of increasing resistance of many bacteria. They are mainly used to treat acute nonobstructive urinary tract infections.

Side effects are numerous and sometimes serious, and can include:

Rash, pruritis, dermatitis, and photosensitivity
Nausea, vomiting, and diarrhea
High fever, headache, stomatitis, and conjunctivitis
Blood dyscracias
Hepatic toxicity with jaundice
Renal damage with crystalluria and hematuria
Hypersensitivity reactions, which can be fatal
Orange urine with Azulfidine and Azo Gantanol

Contraindications include:

Impaired hepatic function
Impaired renal function
Blood dyscracias
Severe allergies or asthma
Pregnancy or lactation

Interactions include:

Potentiation of anticoagulants and hypoglycemics
Antagonism of local anesthetics (e.g., procaine may inhibit antibacterial action of sulfa), and digitalis and phenytoin (Dilantin; sulfonamides may inhibit action)

PATIENT EDUCATION

Patients should be instructed regarding:

Importance of drinking large amounts of fluid to prevent crystalluria
Discontinuance of sulfa at first sign of rash
Reporting any side effects to physician immediately
Avoiding exposure to sunlight
Ingestion of sulfa with food, which delays, but does not reduce, absorption of the drug
Orange urine with Azulfidine and Azo Gantanol (contain pyridium)

Urinary Anti-infectives

Urinary anti-infectives are usually bacteriostatic instead of bactericidal in action. Nitrofurantoin (Furadantin and Macrodantin) are the most commonly used for initial or recurrent urinary tract infections caused by susceptible organisms. Treatment must continue for an adequate period of time to be effective and minimize recurrence of infection.

Side effects can include:

Nausea and vomiting, which are less frequent if taken with milk
Numbness and weakness of lower extremities
Headache, dizziness, and weakness (rare)
Respiratory distress with prolonged use
Brown urine
Anemia

TABLE 13.3. ANTI-INFECTIVE AGENTS: ANTIVIRALS, SULFONAMIDES, AND URINARY ANTI-INFECTIVES

Generic Name	Trade Name	Dosage
Antiviral		
acyclovir	Zovirax	Oint applied q3h × 6 qd 7 days IV 5 mg/kg body weight q8h
Sulfonamides		
sulfasalazine	Azulfidine	Tab, suspension 1–2 g qid in divided doses
sulfasoxazole	Gantrisin	Tab, creams, IV, IM 2–4 g daily in divided doses
co-trimoxazole	Septra, Bactrim	Tab, suspension, IV 160 mg q12h
Urinary Anti-infective		
nitrofurantoin	Macrodantin, Furadantin	Cap, tab, suspension, IV 50–100 mg qid

Contraindications or *caution* applies to:

Renal impairment
Anemia
Diabetes
Electrolyte abnormalities
Asthma
Pregnancy and lactation

Interactions (antagonistic) with:

Benemid and magnesium
Antacids, decreasing the effectiveness of these drugs

PATIENT EDUCATION

Patients should be instructed regarding:

Importance of taking medication for required number of days and follow-up urine culture
Reporting side effects
Taking medication with milk or food to reduce incidence of nausea and vomiting
Avoiding antacids

See Table 13.3 for a summary of the antivirals, sulfonamides, and urinary anti-infectives.

PATIENT EDUCATION

Patients taking antibiotics should be instructed regarding:

Unless directed otherwise, taking all antibiotics with a full glass of water on empty stomach, at least 1 h before meals and 3 h after meals
Not taking with fruit juice
Not taking with antacids
Not taking with alcohol
If side effects occur, discontinuing medication and consulting the physician or pharmacist
Reporting rash, swelling, or breathing difficulty to the physician *immediately*
Taking all antibiotics at prescribed times to maintain blood levels
Taking entire prescription *completely*; *not* discontinuing when symptoms of infection disappear
Not taking any other medications, prescription, or over-the-counter drugs at the same time as antibiotics without checking first with the physician or pharmacist regarding interactions

Anti-infective Drugs

List the drugs according to category and complete all columns. Learn generic or trade names as specified by instructor.

CLASSIFICATIONS AND DRUGS	PURPOSE	SIDE EFFECTS	CONTRAINDICATIONS OR CAUTIONS	PATIENT EDUCATION
Aminoglycosides 1. 2. 3.				
Cephalosporins 1. 2.				
Chloramphenicol 1.				
Penicillins 1. 2. 3. 4.				
Tetracyclines 1. 2. 3.				

CLASSIFICATIONS AND DRUGS	PURPOSE	SIDE EFFECTS	CONTRAINDICATIONS OR CAUTIONS	PATIENT EDUCATION
Erythromycins 1.				
Antifungals 1. 2. 3.				
Anti-TB 1. 2. 3.				
Antiviral 1.				
Sulfonamides 1. 2. 3.				
Urinary Anti-infectives 1. 2.				

14

Eye Medications

OBJECTIVES

Upon completion of this chapter, the student will be able to:

1. Define mydriatic, miotic, and cycloplegic.
2. Demonstrate the administration technique for instillation of ophthalmic medication to reduce systemic absorption.
3. List uses for each category of ophthalmic medication.
4. Identify side effects, contraindications, and interactions for each category of ophthalmic medication.
5. Explain appropriate patient education necessary for each category of eye medication.

Medications for the eye can be classified into five categories: anti-infectives, anti-inflammatory agents, antiglaucoma agents, mydriatics, and local anesthetics.

Anti-infectives

Many anti-infective ophthalmic topical ointments and solutions are available for treatment of superficial infections of the eye caused by susceptible organisms. It is important to determine the causative organism so that the appropriate medication is used.

Side effects can include hypersensitivity reactions including conjunctivitis, burning, rash, and urticaria in allergic persons

Contraindications apply to anyone allergic to the drug.

Interactions may occur with corticosteroids, which can accelerate the spread of infection.

PATIENT EDUCATION

Patients should be instructed regarding:

Careful instillation into the lower conjunctival sac to avoid contamination of the tip of the dropper or ointment tube

Possible hypersensitivity reactions in patients with allergies of any kind

Discontinuance of the medication and reporting immediately to a physician any signs of sensitivity (e.g., burning and itching)

Careful hand washing to prevent spread of infection to other eye or other persons

---

Anti-inflammatory Agents

Anti-inflammatory ophthalmic agents are used to relieve inflammation of the eye or conjunctiva in allergic reactions, burns, or irritation from foreign substances. Various forms of the corticosteroids are also useful in the acute stages of eye injury to prevent scarring but are not used for extended periods because of the danger of masking the symptoms of infection or slowing the healing process. Application of ophthalmic corticosteroids topically does not generally cause systemic effects. However, systemic absorption can be minimized by gentle pressure on the inner canthus of the eye following instillation of corticosteroid ophthalmic drops or ointment.

Side effects of corticosteroids can include:

Increased intraocular pressure (depends on dose, frequency, and length of treatment)

Reduced resistance to bacteria, virus, or fungus

Delayed healing of wounds

Stinging or burning

TABLE 14.1. ANTI-INFLAMMATORY OPHTHALMIC DRUGS

Generic Name	Trade Name	Dosage
corticosteroid	Decadron	Ointment, sol, 0.05%–0.1%
	Hydrocortone	Ointment, suspension

Contraindications or extreme caution applies to:

Acute bacterial, viral, or fungal infections
Primary open-angle glaucoma
Diabetes
Pregnancy
Prolonged use

PATIENT EDUCATION

Patients should be instructed regarding:

Lowered resistance to infection
Administration (i.e., pressure on tear duct at inner corner to reduce systemic absorption)

See Table 14.1 for a summary of anti-inflammatory ophthalmic drugs.

Antiglaucoma Agents

Glaucoma is an abnormal condition of the eye in which there is increased pressure within the eye due to obstruction of the outflow of aqueous humor. There are two main types of glaucoma:

1. *Acute (angle-closure) glaucoma.* Characterized by a sudden onset of pain, blurred vision, and a dilated pupil. If untreated, blindness can result in a few days. **Treatment** consists of miotics (e.g., pilocarpine), osmotic agents (e.g., mannitol), carbonic inhibitors (e.g. Diamox) and surgery to open a pathway for release of aqueous humor.

2. *Chronic (open-angle) glaucoma.* Much more common, often bilateral, and develops slowly over a period of years with few symptoms except a gradual loss of peripheral vision and possibly blurred vision. Halos around lights and central blindness are late manifestations. *Treatment* consists of miotics, carbonic anhydrase inhibitors, and a local beta-adrenergic blocker, such as timolol (Timoptic) eye drops; sometimes epinephrine eye drops are given *with the miotics.* (**Note:** epinephrine ophthalmic drops are *contraindicated in angle-closure glaucoma.*)

Antiglaucoma drugs, given to lower intraocular pressure, can be divided into four main categories based on their mode of action:

1. *Carbonic anhydrase inhibitors.* Act by decreasing the formation of aqueous humor.
2. *Miotics.* Act by increasing the aqueous outflow.
3. *Timolol.* Lowers intraocular pressure by acting as a beta-adrenergic blocker.
4. *Epinephrine ophthalmic drops.* Sometimes given to augment miotics.

CARBONIC ANHYDRASE INHIBITORS

Carbonic anhydrase inhibitors such as acetazolamide (Diamox) reduce the hydrogen and bicarbonate ions and have a diuretic effect. Acetazolamide (Diamox) is administered orally, in the treatment of open-angle glaucoma or short-term preoperatively, to reduce intraocular pressure in angle-closure glaucoma.

Side effects, infrequent and usually dose related, can include:

Nausea, vomiting, diarrhea, and constipation
Thirst and dry mouth
Drowsiness, fatigue, and vertigo
Numbness, muscular weakness, and tingling with high doses
Blood dyscracias
Hepatic and renal disorders

Contraindications or caution applies to:

Chronic obstructive pulmonary disease (COPD)
Diabetes
Hepatic and renal disorders
Pregnancy

Interactions are frequent because of increasing or decreasing excretion of other drugs and can include:

Decreased effects of lithium, phenobarbital, salicylates, and hypoglycemics
Increased effects of procaine, quinidine, amphetamines, and other diuretics
Hypokalemia with thiazides and corticosteroids

PATIENT EDUCATION

Patients should be instructed regarding:

Reporting side effects and response to the physician for appropriate dosage regulation
Importance of follow-up with the physician
Checking with the physician regarding dosage before taking any other medication

MIOTICS

Miotics are medications that cause the pupil to contract. Miotics reduce intraocular pressure by increasing the aqueous outflow. They act by contracting the ciliary muscle. Miotics (e.g., pilocarpine), are used in the treatment of open-angle glaucoma or in short-term treatment of angle-closure glaucoma before surgery. Pilocarpine is also used after ophthalmic examinations in glaucoma patients to *constrict the pupil* and counteract the *mydriatic* (pupil-dilating) effect.

Side effects can include:

Blurred vision and myopia
Twitching, stinging, and burning
Ocular pain and headache
Photophobia and poor vision in dim light
Aggravation of inflammatory processes
Hypersensitivity, conjunctivitis, and dermatitis with physostigmine

Systemic effects with frequent or prolonged use can include:

Nausea, vomiting, and diarrhea
Increased lacrimation and salivation

Contraindications or caution applies to:

Angle-closure glaucoma
History of retinal detachment
Acute inflammatory processes
Soft lenses in place
Corneal abrasion

Interactions may occur with:

Topical epinephrine, timolol, and acetazolamid, which increase miotic effect
Some anesthetics, which are potentiated by some miotics

PATIENT EDUCATION

Patients should be instructed regarding:

Administration by closing tear duct after instillation
Reporting side effects to the physician for possible dosage adjustment
Administration at bedtime to reduce side effects
Not driving at night

TIMOLOL

Timolol acts as a beta-adrenergic blocker. It is used topically to lower intraocular pressure in open-angle glaucoma.

Side effects are infrequent but may include:

Ocular irritation and conjunctivitis
Aggravation of *preexisting* cardiovascular or pulmonary disorders, which may cause bradycardia, hypotension and vertigo, or bronchospasm

Contraindications or extreme caution applies to:

Bradycardia and heart block
Patients receiving oral beta-blocker drugs
Asthma and COPD
Children, pregnancy, and lactation

Interactions may occur with:

Other antiglaucoma drugs to help lower intraocular pressure
Oral beta blockers to increase chances of hypotension, bradycardia, and heart block

---

PATIENT EDUCATION

Patients should be instructed regarding:

Administration by closing tear duct after instillation to reduce systemic effects
Caution in patients with cardiac or pulmonary disorders or who are taking oral beta blockers
Importance of regular eye examinations
Continuous use of medications for glaucoma
When administering more than one ophthalmic medication, allowing time interval (at least 5 min) between medications

---

EPINEPHRINE

Epinephrine has a mydriatic effect in patients with open-angle glaucoma but is ineffective as a mydriatic in normal eyes, except during surgery. Epinephrine is sometimes combined with miotics in the treatment of open-angle glaucoma (not for angle-closure glaucoma). Epinephrine augments the action of miotics.

Side effects are frequent with topical application of epinephrine and include:

Burning, stinging, pain, and headache
Blurred vision and photophobia
Allergic reactions (e.g., dermatitis and edema)
Systemic effects, including palpitation, tachycardia, and tremor

Contraindications or extreme caution applies to:

Cardiac disorders and hypertension
Diabetes

Thyroid disorders

Cerebral arteriosclerosis

PATIENT EDUCATION

Patients should be instructed regarding reporting side effects to the physician immediately.

See Table 14.2 for a summary of ophthalmic drugs for glaucoma.

TABLE 14.2. OPHTHALMIC DRUGS FOR GLAUCOMA

Generic Name	Trade Name	Dosage	Comments
Carbonic Anhydrase Inhibitor			
acetazolamide	Diamox	Cap, tab, IV, IM 250–500 mg qd or bid	
Miotics[a]			
pilocarpine	Isopto Carpine	Ophthalmic sol, 0.25%–10%[b]	
physostigmine	Isopto Eserine	Ophthalmic sol, oint, 0.25%–0.5%	
Beta-Adrenergic Blocker			
timolol	Timoptic	Ophthalmic sol, 0.25% or 0.5%	
Mydriatic			
epinephrine	Epifrin	Ophthalmic sol, 0.1%–2%	In combination with miotics for open-angle glaucoma only

[a]Contract the pupil.
[b]Wide variation in strengths available. Check carefully for correct percentage.

Mydriatics

Mydriatics (e.g., atropine) are used to *dilate the pupil* for ophthalmic examinations. Atropine also acts as a *cycloplegic* (paralyzes the muscles of accommodation for eye examinations).

Side effects of atropine, more likely in geriatric patients, may include:

Increased intraocular pressure

Local irritation

Blurred vision

Flushing, dryness of skin, and fever

Confusion

Contraindications apply to:

Angle-closure glaucoma

Infants

PATIENT EDUCATION

Patients should be instructed regarding:

Administration by closing tear duct after instillation
Aseptic technique to prevent contamination of medicine

Epinephrine has a mydriatic effect in patients with open-angle glaucoma and also lowers intraocular pressure but is ineffective as a mydriatic in normal eyes, except during surgery. For side effects, contraindications, and patient education see "Epinephrine" under "Anti-Glaucoma Agents."

See Table 14.3 for a summary of the mydriatics.

TABLE 14.3. MYDRIATICS AND LOCAL ANESTHETICS FOR THE EYE

Generic Name	Trade Name	Dosage	Comments
Mydriatics[a]			
atropine	Atropine	Oint, 0.5%–1% Ophthalmic sol, 0.5%–3%[b]	
epinephrine	Epifrin	Ophthalmic sol, 0.1%–2%	In combination with miotics for open-angle glaucoma only
Local Anesthetics			
tetracaine	Pontocaine	Oint or sol, 0.5%	

[a]Dilate the pupil.
[b]Wide variations in strengths available. Check carefully for correct percentage.

Local Anesthetics

Local ophthalmic anesthetics, such as tetracaine (*Pontocaine*), are applied topically to the eye for minor surgical procedures, removal of foreign bodies, or painful injury.

Side effects are rare except with prolonged use but may include hypersensitivity reactions such as anaphylaxis in those allergic to the "-caine" local anesthetics.

Contraindicated for prolonged use.

PATIENT EDUCATION

Patients should be instructed regarding:

Necessity of wearing an eye patch after use of pontocaine because of loss of blink reflex
Avoidance of touching or rubbing the eye until the anesthesia has worn off

---

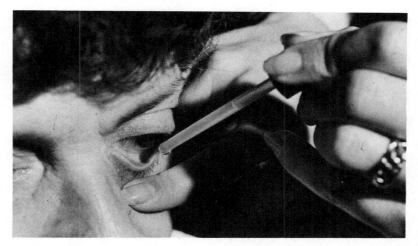

Figure 14.1   *Instilling eye medication. Ophthalmic solution is dropped inside lower eyelid.*

PATIENT EDUCATION

Patients taking ophthalmic medications, should be instructed regarding:

Instillation of the *correct number of drops* or amount of ointment into the conjunctival sac (Fig. 14.1)

Closing the eye gently so as not to squeeze the medication out

Applying gentle pressure to inner canthus after instillation to minimize systemic effects (Fig. 14.2)

Making certain the correct medication and correct percent solution are used as prescribed

Proper aseptic technique to prevent contamination of the other eye, the dropper, or the ointment tube

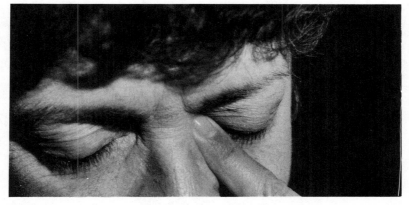

Figure 14.2   *Gentle pressure on the inner canthus following administration of ophthalmic medications. Systemic absorption is thus minimized with medications such as corticosteroids, miotics, and mydriatics.*

WORKSHEET FOR CHAPTER 14

Eye Medications

List the drugs according to category and complete all columns. Learn generic or trade names as specified by instructor.

CLASSIFICATIONS AND DRUGS	PURPOSE	SIDE EFFECTS	CONTRAINDICATIONS OR CAUTIONS	PATIENT EDUCATION
Anti-inflammatory 1.				
Antiglaucoma 1.				
Miotics 1. 2.				
Beta-Adrenergic Blocker 1.				
Mydriatics 1. 2.				
Local Anesthetic 1.				

15

Urinary System Drugs

OBJECTIVES

Upon completion of this chapter, the student will be able to:

1. Compare and contrast the four types of diuretics for uses, side effects, cautions, and interactions and give examples of each type.
2. Define hypokalemia, hyperkalemia, calculus, diuretic, and uricosuric.
3. Describe two interactions of other medications with Benemid.
4. Identify one medication given for chronic gout that is not uricosuric and one that is.
5. Explain the role of certain antispasmodics used to reduce contractions of the urinary bladder.
6. Identify the actions of phenazopyridine (Urecholine) and bethanechol (Pyridium).
7. Describe appropriate patient education for all medications listed in this chapter.

Diuretics

The most commonly used drugs influencing function of the urinary tract are the diuretics, which increase urine excretion. Diuretics are divided into four categories according to their action: thiazides, potent nonthiazide diuretics, potassium-sparing diuretics, and osmotic agents. The type of diuretic used is determined by the condition of the patient.

THIAZIDES

Thiazides are the most frequently used type of diuretic, increasing excretion of water, sodium, chloride, and potassium. An example is chlorothiazide (Diuril).

Uses of the thiazides include treatment of:

Edema from many causes (e.g., heart failure and cirrhosis)
Hypertension (blood pressure is lowered by direct arterial dilation, as well as by decreasing fluid retention)
Prophylaxis of calculus (stone) formation in those with hypercalciuria (excess calcium in the urine)

Side effects of the thiazides may include:

Hypokalemia (excess potassium depletion), which may lead to cardiac arrhythmias
Muscle weakness or spasm
GI reactions (e.g., anorexia, nausea, vomiting, diarrhea, and cramping)
Postural hypotension, vertigo, and headache
Fatigue, weakness, and lethargy
Skin conditions (e.g., rash and photosensitivity; rare)
Hyperglycemia and increased uric acid

Contraindications or caution applies to:

Diabetes (may cause hyperglycemia and glycosuria)
History of gout (increased uric acid level)
Severe renal disease
Impaired liver function
Prolonged use (periodic serum electrolyte checks indicated, and potassium supplements recommended to prevent hypokalemia)

Interactions may occur with:

Corticosteroids to increase potassium loss
Lithium, to cause lithium intoxication
Hypotensive agents, which potentiate blood pressure decrease

Probenecid (Benemid), to block uric acid excretion

. Alcohol, barbiturates, and opiates to increase postural hypotension

---

PATIENT EDUCATION

Patients should be instructed regarding:

Diet including potassium-rich foods (e.g., citrus fruits and bananas) or potassium supplements (check with the physician first)

If diuretic prescribed for hypertension, a low-sodium diet (may be prescribed by the physician)

Notifying the physician of persistent or severe side effects

Administration with food (to reduce gastric irritation) at least 6 h before bedtime

Rising slowly from reclining position to counteract postural hypotension

Limitation of alcohol

POTENT NONTHIAZIDE DIURETICS

Potent diuretics such as furosemide (Lasix) and ethacrynic acid (Edecrin) are not thiazides but act in a similar way to increase excretion of water, sodium, chloride, and potassium. Their action is more rapid and effective than that of the thiazides, with a greater diuresis.

Uses of potent nonthiazides such as furosemide (Lasix) and ethacrynic acid (Edecrin), include treatment of:

Congestive heart failure

Pulmonary edema

Ascites caused by malignancy

Hypertension (if thiazides ineffective, furosemide or ethacrynic acid sometimes combined with other antihypertensives)

Side effects of furosemide and ethacrynic acid may include:

Fluid and electrolyte imbalance with dehydration

Hypokalemia with weakness and vertigo (potassium supplements indicated especially for cardiac patients to prevent arrhythmias)

Hypotension (close blood pressure checks required)

GI effects, including anorexia, nausea, vomiting, diarrhea, and abdominal pain

Hyperglycemia and increased uric acid

Blood dyscrasias with prolonged use

Tinnitus, hearing impairment, and blurred vision

Rash, urticaria, pruritis, and photosensitivity

Allergic reactions to furosemide in those allergic to sulfa, since furosemide is a *sulfonamide*

Headache, muscle cramps, and mental confusion

Contraindications or caution applies to:

Cirrhosis and other liver disease
Kidney impairment
Alkalosis and dehydration
Digitalized patients (cardiac arrhythmias possible unless potassium supplemented)
Diabetes
History of gout
Pregnancy and lactation

Interactions of furosemide and ethacrynic acid are similar to those of the thiazides (see thiazide interactions):

Corticosteroids
Lithium
Hypotensive agents
Probenecid
Alcohol, barbiturates, and opiates

Additional interactions of furosemide and ethacrynic acid may include:

Aminoglycosides to increase chance of deafness
Coumadin with ethacrynic acid to potentiate anticoagulant effect
Indomethacin to antagonize the effect of furosemide in lowering blood pressure
Salicylates with furosemide to increase chance of salicylate toxicity
Anticonvulsants (e.g., phenytoin) to reduce the diuretic effect of furosemide

---

PATIENT EDUCATION

Patients should be instructed regarding the same information as patients taking thiazides:

Dietary or other potassium supplements as prescribed
Notifying the physician of side effects
Taking with food before 6 P.M.
Rising slowly from reclining position
Avoiding alcohol

Patients taking furosemide or ethacrynic acid should also be instructed regarding:

Limiting exposure to sunlight
Not taking any other prescribed or over-the-counter drugs without consulting the physician first
Reporting any side effects, especially rash

POTASSIUM-SPARING DIURETICS

Potassium-sparing diuretics such as spironolactone (Aldactone) and triamterene (Dyrenium), are sometimes administered under conditions in which potassium depletion can be dangerous. Potassium-sparing diuretics also counteract the increased glucose and uric acid levels associated with thiazide diuretic therapy.

Potassium-sparing diuretics are seldom used alone, but are usually combined with thiazide diuretics to increase the diuretic and hypotensive effects and to reduce the danger of hyperkalemia (excessive potassium retention). When combination products (e.g., Aldactazide or Dyazide) are given, supplemental potassium is usually *not* indicated, but this varies with individual circumstances and other medications taken concomitantly. Periodic serum electrolyte checks are indicated.

Side effects of potassium-saving diuretics are usually mild and respond to withdrawal of the the drug, but may include:

Hyperkalemia (especially with potassium supplements), which may lead to cardiac arrhythmias
Dehydration or weakness
GI symptoms, including nausea, vomiting, and diarrhea
Fatigue, lethargy, and profound weight loss
Hypotension

Caution is indicated in patients with:

Renal insufficiency
Cirrhosis and other liver disease

Interactions may occur with:

Potassium supplements to cause hyperkalemia
Beta blockers to potentiate blocking effects
Penicillin G potassium to cause hyperkalemia

PATIENT EDUCATION

Patients should be instructed regarding:

Avoidance of potassium-rich foods and salt substitutes
Reporting signs of excessive dehydration (e.g., dry mouth, drowsiness, lethargy, and fever)
Reporting GI symptoms (e.g., nausea, vomiting, and diarrhea)
Reporting persistent headache and mental confusion
Monitoring weight and reporting sudden, excessive weight loss
Rising slowly from reclining position
Taking medications after meals

OSMOTIC AGENTS

Osmotic agents (e.g., mannitol and urea) are most frequently used to reduce intracranial or intraocular pressure. Mannitol has also been used to prevent and/or treat acute renal failure and during certain cardiovascular surgery. Mannitol is also used alone or with other diuretics to promote excretions of toxins in cases of drug poisoning.

Side effects can include:

Fluid and electrolyte imbalance
CNS symptoms, including headache, vertigo, mental confusion, nausea, and vomiting
Tachycardia, hypertension, and hypotension
Allergic reactions

Extreme caution is indicated, and kidney and cardiovascular function should be evaluated before administration of these drugs to anyone with:

Kidney failure
Cardiovascular disease
Liver disease
Pregnancy and lactation

Interactions may occur with mannitol to increase urinary excretion of other drugs. Blood levels of drugs such as lithium are lowered as a result.

PATIENT EDUCATION

Patients should be instructed regarding side effects to be reported to the physician immediately. The patient should be reassured that osmotic agents are always given under close medical supervision and serum electrolytes will be monitored frequently by blood tests to detect adverse reactions.

See Table 15.1 for a summary of drugs for diuresis.

Medications for Gout

Medications to treat gout include uricosuric agents and allopurinol, which lowers uric acid levels.

URICOSURIC AGENTS

Uricosuric agents, such as probenecid (Benemid), act on the kidney by blocking reabsorption and promoting urinary excretion of uric acid. This type of drug is

TABLE 15.1. DRUGS FOR DIURESIS

Generic Name	Trade Name	Dosage
Thiazide Diuretics		
chlorothiazide	Diuril	500 mg–2 g qd PO
hydrochlorothiazide	Esidrex	25–50 mg bid or tid
Potent Nonthiazide Diuretics		
ethacrynic acid	Edecrin	50–100 mg qd or bid
furosemide	Lasix	20–80 mg qd
		20–40 mg IM or IV
Potassium-Sparing Diuretics		
spironolactone	Aldactone	50–100 mg qd
triamterene	Dyrenium	100 mg bid pc
Combination Potassium-Sparing and Thiazide Diuretics		
	Aldactazide	50–100 mg qd
	Dyazide	1 cap bid
Osmotic Agents		
mannitol	Osmitrol	Parenteral only, dose varies with condition
urea	Ureaphil	Injection usually, dose varies with condition

used in the treatment of *chronic* cases of gout and frequent disabling attacks of gouty arthritis. However, the uricosuric agents have no analgesic or anti-inflammatory activity and are therefore *not* effective in the treatment of acute gout.

Probenecid is sometimes given with penicillin to potentiate the level of the antibiotic in the blood.

Side effects of probenecid are rare but may include:

Headache
Nausea and vomiting
Kidney stones and renal colic

Contraindications apply to patients with:

History of uric acid kidney stones
History of peptic ulcer
Renal impairment

Interactions may occur with:

Penicillins and cephalosporins, which potentiate antibiotic effect
Oral hypoglycemics, which could cause hypoglycemia through potentiation
Salicylates, which antagonize uricosuric action

PATIENT EDUCATION

Patients should be instructed regarding:

Drinking large amounts of fluid
Avoiding taking any aspirin products
Taking other medications at the same time only with physician's order
Taking medications with food

ALLOPURINOL

Allopurinol (Zyloprim) is another medication, not a uricosuric, used to treat chronic gout. This drug acts by decreasing serum and urine levels of uric acid. It has no analgesic or anti-inflammatory activity, and therefore is *not* effective in the treatment of acute gout. *Note:* The drug of choice for acute cases of gout or gouty arthritis is *colchicine*, which is discussed in Chapter 21.

Allopurinol is also used for the prevention of renal calculi in patients with a history of frequent stone formation.

Side effects can include:

Rash
Allergic reactions, including fever, chills, nausea, vomiting, diarrhea, drowsiness, and vertigo

Contraindications or caution applies to:

Impaired renal function
History of hypersensitivity reactions
Liver disease
Pregnancy and lactation

Interactions may occur with:

Antineoplastic drug, which are potentiated
Alcohol and diuretics, which increase serum urate concentrations

---

PATIENT EDUCATION

Patients should be instructed regarding:

Drinking large quantities of fluid
Taking medication after meals
Stopping medication and reporting rash to physician immediately
Avoiding alcohol, which increases uric acid
Avoiding other medications unless prescribed by physician

Antispasmodics

Antispasmodics, which are anticholinergic in action (blocking parasympathetic nerve impulses), are used to reduce the strength and frequency of contractions of the urinary bladder. Antispasmodics, such as methantheline (Banthine), are used to increase the bladder capacity in patients with neurogenic bladder, incontinence, or functional enuresis.

Side effects are anticholinergic in action and can include:

Drying of all secretions
Drowsiness and dizziness
Urinary retention
Constipation
Blurred vision (dilated pupils)

PATIENT EDUCATION

Patients should be instructed regarding:

Reporting side effects that are troublesome for possible dosage adjustment
Reporting effectiveness (relief of spasm)
Using caution driving or operating machinery

Analgesics

Phenazopyridine (Pyridium) is an analgesic or local anesthetic for urinary tract mucosa. It is used to relieve burning, pain, discomfort, and urgency associated with cystitis; with procedures causing irritation to the lower urinary tract, such as cystoscopy and surgery; or with trauma.

Phenazopyridine is used *only for symptomatic relief* and is not a substitute for treatment of causative conditions. For treatment of urinary tract infections, anti-infective medication is required. See Chapter 13.

Side effects are rare for the most part but can include:

Headache or vertigo
Mild GI disturbances
Orange-red urine (common)

Contraindications include:

Impaired kidney function
Severe hepatitis

Phenazopyridine may interfere with various urine, kidney function, or liver function tests.

PATIENT EDUCATION

Patients should be instructed regarding color change of urine to orange-red, which may stain fabric.

Phenazopyridine is only temporarily effective against discomfort in the lower urinary tract and is *not* effective against infection. The cause of the discomfort must be determined by examination of urine culture, and appropriate therapy, such as surgery or anti-infective medication, may be given to correct the condition.

Cholinergics

Bethanechol (Urecholine) is a cholinergic drug, stimulating parasympathetic nerves, to bring about contraction of the urinary bladder in cases of *nonobstructive* urinary retention. It has been called the "pharmacological catheterization."

Side effects are cholinergic in action and usually dose related, and can include:

GI cramping, diarrhea, nausea, and vomiting
Sweating and salivation
Headache and bronchial constriction
Tachycardia

Contraindications include:

Obstruction of the GI or urinary tract
Hyperthyroidism
Peptic ulcer
Asthma
Cardiovascular disease
Pregnancy and lactation

Interactions may occur with:

Other cholinergic or anticholinesterase agents (e.g., neostigmine) administered concomitantly, which can potentiate effects, with increased possibility of toxicity
Beta blockers, which may result in critical fall in blood pressure
Quinidine or procainamide, which antagonize cholinergic effect
Atropine, which antagonizes cholinergic effect (antidote in cases of cholinergic toxicity)

TABLE 15.2. OTHER DRUGS AFFECTING THE URINARY TRACT

Generic Name	Trade Name	Dosage
Uricosuric Agents		
probenecid	Benemid	250–500 mg bid
sulfinpyrazone	Anturane	100–100 mg bid
Antigout Medication		
allopurinol	Zyloprim	
Antispasmodics		
methantheline	Banthine	50–100 mg qid
propantheline	Pro-Banthine	15–30 mg qid
Analgesic		
phenazopyridine	Pyridium	200 mg tid pc
Cholinergic[a]		
bethanecol	Urecholine	PO or SC, *never* IM or IV Dose according to condition

[a]For bladder contraction.

PATIENT EDUCATION

Patients should be instructed regarding:

Reporting any unpleasant or persistent side effects
Avoiding taking other medications at same time without permission of physician
Recording amount and frequency of urination if requested by physician

---

WORKSHEET FOR CHAPTER 15

Urinary System Drugs

List the drugs according to category and complete all columns. Learn generic or trade names as specified by instructor.

CLASSIFICATIONS AND DRUGS	PURPOSE	SIDE EFFECTS	CONTRAINDICATIONS OR CAUTIONS	PATIENT EDUCATION
Thiazides 1. 2.				
Potent Nonthiazide Diuretics 1. 2.				
Potassium-Sparing Diuretics 1. 2.				
Combination Potassium-Sparing and Thiazide Diuretics 1. 2.				
Osmotic Agents 1.				
Uricosuric Agents 1.				

CLASSIFICATIONS AND DRUGS	PURPOSE	SIDE EFFECTS	CONTRAINDICATIONS OR CAUTIONS	PATIENT EDUCATION
Antigout Medications				
1.				
Antispasmodics				
1.				
2.				
Analgesic				
1.				
Cholinergic				
1.				

16

Gastrointestinal Drugs

OBJECTIVES

Upon completion of this chapter, the student will be able to:

1. Define antiflatulent, antiemetic, laxative, and cathartic.
2. Describe side effects, contraindications, and interactions of antacids, anti-ulcer agents, antidiarrhea agents, antiflatulents, cathartics and laxatives, and antiemetics.
3. Compare and contrast the five types of laxatives according to use, side effects, contraindications, and interactions.
4. Identify examples of drugs from each of the six categories of gastrointestinal drugs.
5. Explain important patient education for each category of gastrointestinal drugs.

Gastrointestinal drugs can be divided into six categories based on the action: antacids, antiulcer agents, antidiarrhea agents, antiflatulents, laxatives and cathartics, and antiemetics.

Antacids

Antacids act by partially *neutralizing* gastric hydrochloric acid and are widely available in many over-the-counter preparations for the relief of indigestion, heartburn, and sour stomach. Antacids are also prescribed at times, (between meals and at hour of sleep) to help relieve pain and promote the healing of gastric and duodenal ulcers. Other antiulcer agents are discussed later in this chapter.

Antacid products may contain aluminum, calcium carbonate, or magnesium, either individually or in combination. Most antacids also contain sodium. Sodium bicarbonate alone is not recommended because of flatulence, metabolic alkalosis, and electrolyte imbalance with prolonged use.

Side effects of antacids may include:

Constipation (with aluminum or calcium carbonate antacids)
Diarrhea (with magnesium antacids)
Acid rebound (with calcium carbonate)
Electrolyte imbalance
Urinary calculi and renal complications
Osteoporosis (with aluminum antacids)
Belching and flatulence (with calcium carbonate and sodium bicarbonate)

Contraindications or extreme caution applies to:

Congestive heart failure
Renal pathology or history of renal calculi
Cirrhosis of the liver or edema
Dehydration or electrolyte imbalance

PATIENT EDUCATION

Patients should be instructed regarding:

Avoiding prolonged use (no longer than 2 weeks) of OTC antacids without medical supervision because of the danger of masking symptoms of GI bleeding or GI malignancy

Avoiding the use of antacids at the same time as any other medication because of many interactions

Avoiding the use of antacids entirely if patient has cardiac, renal, or liver disease or fluid retention

---

Interactions with almost any other drug administered concurrently can alter the effectiveness of the other drugs. Therefore, antacids should *not be* taken within 2 hours of any other drug. With the following drugs, antacids may *decrease* effectiveness of the drug:

Antibiotics, especially tetracyclines
Digoxin, indomethacin, and iron
Salicylates and isoniazid

Antacids with the following drugs may *increase* action and precipitate side effects:

Coumarin, which increases bleeding
Diazepam, which increases sedation
Amphetamines and quinidine, which increase cardiac irregularities

Antiulcer Agents

Newer anti-ulcer agents *reduce gastric acid secretion* by acting as *histamine$_2$ receptor antagonists.* Two of the drugs in this category, cimetidine (Tagamet) and ranitidine (Zantac), are used in the treatment of duodenal ulcers, gastric ulcers, GI hypersecretory conditions, and upper GI bleeding or esophagitis.

Side effects, usually transient and dose-related, can include:

Diarrhea, dizziness, rash, and headache
Mild gynecomastia
Mental confusion (especially in the elderly)

PATIENT EDUCATION

Patients should be instructed regarding:

Avoidance of cigarette smoking, which seems to decrease the effectiveness of ranitidine in the healing of duodenal ulcers

Importance of close communication with the physician for possible dosage regulation of other medications taken at the same time

Structuring of environment to reduce stress factors and decrease tension in order to facilitate healing of ulcers and reduce gastric motility and hypersecretion, as an adjunct to drug therapy

Not taking antacids, if ordered, within 2 h of taking cimetidine or ranitidine

Taking medications on a regular basis and avoiding abrupt withdrawal, which could lead to rebound hypersecretion of gastric acid

---

Contraindications or extreme caution applies to:

Impaired renal function
Liver dysfunction
Children, pregnancy, and lactation

Interactions may occur with increased blood concentrations of:

Coumarin anticoagulants
Phenytoin
Propranolol
Diazepam
Lidocaine
Theophyllin

Antidiarrhea Agents

Antidiarrhea agents act in various ways to reduce the number of loose stools.

KAOLIN AND PECTIN

Kaolin and pectin preparations (e.g., Kaopectate) act as *adsorbents and protectants* to achieve a drying effect (i.e., decrease fluidity of stools).

Side effects are relatively nonexistant, other than transient constipation on occasion.

PATIENT EDUCATION

Patients should be instructed regarding:

Avoiding self-medication for longer than 48 h or if fever develops without consulting a physician

Diet of a bland nature, excluding roughage, and including foods containing natural pectin (e.g., apple without peelings and *without* sugar added to apple)

Adequate fluid intake (especially tea *without* sugar for its astringent effect) to prevent dehydration

Contacting the physician immediately if complications develop or condition worsens

Taking other medications (e.g., antibiotics or digitalis) 2–3 h before or after taking kaolin and pectin products

---

Interactions are possible, such as impaired absorption, when these agents are administered concurrently with such other medications as:

Lincomycin
Digoxin

Contraindications, without medical supervision, may occur in infants and the elderly.

DIPHENOXYLATE WITH ATROPINE

Diphenoxylate with atropine (Lomotil) and loperamide (Imodium) act by *slowing intestinal motility.*

Side effects can include:

With Lomotil, anticholinergic effects (e.g., drying of secretions, blurred vision, urinary retention, lethargy, confusion, or flushing)
With Lomotil and Imodium, abdominal distention, nausea, or vomiting

Contraindications or caution applies to:

Diarrhea caused by infection or poisoning
Young children and pregnancy
Lincomycin-induced colitis

PATIENT EDUCATION

Patients should be instructed regarding:

Bland diet
Adequate fluid intake
Reporting side effects or complications to the physician immediately

---

Antiflatulents

Antiflatulents (e.g., simethicone) are used in the symptomatic treatment of gastric bloating and postoperative gas pains, by helping to break up gas bubbles in the GI tract.
No side effects have been reported.

Contraindications apply to infant colic because of limited information on safety in children.

PATIENT EDUCATION

Patients should be instructed to avoid gas-forming foods (e.g., onions, cabbage, and beans).

See Table 16.1 for a summary of Antacids, Antiulcer Agents, Antidiarrhea Agents, and Antiflatulents.

TABLE 16.1. ANTACIDS, ANTIULCER AGENTS, ANTIDIARRHEA AGENTS, AND ANTIFLATULENTS

Generic Name	Trade Name	Dosage
Antacids		
aluminum	Amphojel	Suspension, 320 mg/5 ml Tabs, 300 mg
calcium carbonate	Alka-2, Tums	Tabs, 500 mg
aluminum-magnesium combinations	Riopan, Maalox, Gelusil, Mylanta	Suspension, tabs, dose varies with product
Antiulcer Agents[a]		
ranitidine	Zantac	150-mg tabs bid
cimetidine	Tagamet	200–300-mg tabs q6h 150–300 mg IM, IV
Antidiarrhea Agents		
diphenoxylate with atropine	Lomotil	Sol or tabs, 2.5–5 mg qid
kaolin and pectin	Kaopectate	Suspension, 45–90 ml after each bowel movement
kaolin, pectin, and belladonna	Donnagel	15 ml q3h PRN, maximum 75 mg total qd
loperamide	Imodium	2-mg caps after each bowel movement, maximum 16 mg total qd
Antiflatulent		
simethicone	Mylicon	Suspension, tabs pc and hs 150–400 mg qd in divided doses

[a]Histamine-receptor antagonists.

Laxatives and Cathartics

Laxatives promote evacuation of the intestine. Included in the laxative category are *cathartics*, or *purgatives*, which promote rapid evacuation of the intestine and alteration of stool consistency. Laxatives can be subdivided into five categories according to their action: bulk-forming laxatives, stool softeners, mineral oil, saline laxatives, and stimulant laxatives.

Many OTC laxatives are self-prescribed and overused by a large portion of the population. Prevention and relief of constipation is better achieved through natural methods (e.g., high-fiber diet, adequate fluid intake, good bowel habits, and exercise).

BULK-FORMING LAXATIVES

Bulk-forming laxatives (e.g., psyllium) are the treatment of choice for simple constipation unrelieved by natural methods. These products are available in powders, flakes, granules, tablets, or liquids and *must be dissolved* according to manufacturers' directions (note label). The usual procedure is to dissolve the product in *one full glass* of water or juice to be taken orally and followed immediately with another glass of fluid. The proper dosage is administered one to three times per day. Laxative effect is usually apparent within 12–24 h.

Contraindications apply to patients with acute abdominal pain, partial bowel obstruction, or dysphagia.

PATIENT EDUCATION

Patients should be instructed regarding dissolving all bulk-forming products completely in one full glass of liquid and following that with another glass of fluid to prevent obstruction.

STOOL SOFTENERS

Stool softeners (e.g., docusate combinations) are another mild form of laxative administered orally. Dosage required to soften stools varies widely depending on the condition and patient response.

Side effects are rare, with occasional mild, transitory GI cramping or rash.

Contraindications include acute abdominal pain or prolonged use (more than 1 week) without medical supervision.

PATIENT EDUCATION

Patients should be instructed regarding:

   Discontinuance with any signs of diarrhea or abdominal pain
   Avoiding use for longer than 1 week without medical supervision
   Interaction with mineral oil, which leads to mucosal irritation

---

MINERAL OIL

Mineral oil may be administered orally in emulsion form for palatability (e.g., Agoral or Petrogalar) and is usually effective in 6–8 h. Mineral oil is sometimes administered rectally as an oil retention enema (60–150 ml).

Side effects may include:

Seepage of oil from rectum, causing anal irritation
Malabsorption of vitamins A, D, E, and K only with prolonged oral use

Contraindications for oral mineral oil include:

Children under 6 years old
Bedridden, debilitated, or geriatric patients
Patients with dysphagia, gastric retention, or hiatal hernia
Pregnancy
Prolonged use
Concomitant use of stool softeners

PATIENT EDUCATION

Patients should be instructed regarding:

Avoiding frequent or prolonged use
Caution with anyone who might have trouble swallowing or who might aspirate the oil

---

SALINE LAXATIVES

Saline laxatives (e.g., milk of magnesia) should be taken only infrequently in single doses. Saline laxatives should *never* be taken on a regular or repeated basis.

Side effects of saline laxatives used for prolonged periods or in overdoses can include:

Electrolyte imbalance
CNS symptoms, including weakness, sedation, and confusion
Edema
Cardiac, renal, and hepatic complications

Contraindications include:

Congestive heart failure
Edema, cirrhosis, or renal disorders
Acute abdominal pain

PATIENT EDUCATION

Patients should be instructed regarding:

  Avoiding saline cathartics with the contraindicated medical disorders
  Avoiding frequent or regular use of saline cathartics

STIMULANT LAXATIVES

Stimulant laxatives (e.g., senna, cascara, phenolphthalein, aloe, and bisacodyl) are cathartic in action, producing strong peristaltic activity, and may also alter intestinal secretions in several ways. Stimulant laxatives are habit forming, and long-term use may result in laxative dependence and loss of normal bowel function. All stimulant laxatives produce some degree of abdominal discomfort. Their use should be confined to conditions in which rapid, thorough emptying of the bowel is required (e.g., before surgical, proctoscopic, sigmoidoscopic, or radiologic examinations, or for emptying the bowel of barium following GI X-rays). Sometimes a combination of oral preparations, suppositories, and/or enemas may be ordered for these purposes.

Side effects are common, especially with frequent use and can include:

Abdominal cramps or discomfort and nausea (frequent)
Rectal and/or colonic irritation with suppositories
Loss of normal bowel function with prolonged use
Electrolyte disturbances with prolonged use
Pink, red, or brown discoloration to urine with aloe, cascara, senna, or
  phenolphthalein

Contraindications or extreme caution applies to:

Acute abdominal pain or abdominal cramping
Ulcerative colitis
Children, pregnancy, and lactation

PATIENT EDUCATION

Patients taking stimulant laxatives should be given strong warnings against frequent or prolonged use because of danger of laxative dependence and loss of normal bowel function.

PATIENT EDUCATION

Patients taking any laxative should be instructed regarding:

High-fiber diet to prevent constipation, including roughage, (e.g., bran and fresh fruits and vegetables)

Adequate fluid intake

Developing good bowel habits (e.g., regular, at an unrushed time of day)

Regular exercise to develop muscle tone

Avoiding any laxative with acute abdominal pain, nausea, vomiting, or fever

Avoiding laxatives if any medical condition is present, unless prescribed by a physician

Use of only the mildest laxatives (e.g., stool softeners) on a short-term, infrequent basis

Reporting any prolonged constipation, if above measures are ineffective, to a physician for investigation

---

Antiemetics

Antiemetics are used in the prevention or treatment of nausea, vomiting, or motion sickness. Many different types of products are available, varying in their actions, the condition treated, and route of administration.

The three antiemetics used most frequently to control nausea and vomiting are Emete-Con, Compazine, and Tigan, which are related to the phenothiazines or antihistamines, discussed in Chapters 20 and 27. These drugs are used for symptomatic relief, and their use must be supplemented by restoration of fluid and electrolyte balance, as well as determination of the cause of vomiting.

For preoperative preventative antiemetic effect or postoperative treatment for nausea and vomiting, a phenothiazine (e.g., Phenergan) is usually the drug of choice.

For treatment of motion sickness, preventive drugs such as dymenhydrinate (Dramamine) or scopolamine are used. For greatest effectiveness, the Transderm-Scop patch is applied behind the ear 4 h before anticipated exposure to motion and is effective up to 72 h. Dramamine is administered orally 30 min before exposure to motion. Both of these drugs are also available for intramuscular injection in patients who have already developed motion sickness.

Side effects of the antiemetics vary with the drug and dosage, but the most common include:

Sedation, drowsiness, vertigo, and confusion

Dry mouth and blurred vision

Extrapyramidal reactions (involuntary movements), especially in children and the elderly

Cardiac arrhythmias (rare)

TABLE 16.2. LAXATIVES AND ANTIEMETICS

Generic Name	Trade Name	Dosage
Laxatives		
Bulk-forming		
psyllium	Metamucil	Powder, 1 tsp, dissolve in full glass of fluid 1–3 × /day; follow with full glass of fluid
Stool softener		
docusate	Surfak, Doxidan, Dialose, Colace	Oral caps, liquid 50–360 mg qd
Mineral oil	Agoral, Kondremul, Petrogalar	15–45 ml PO
Saline laxatives	Milk of Magnesia	300–600-mg tabs 30–60-ml suspension
Stimulant laxatives		
cascara sagrada fluid extract		0.5–1.5-ml single dose
senna	X-prep	7.5-mg or 5-ml single dose
bisacodyl	Dulcolax	5–15 mg tabs 10-mg supp
phenolphthalein	Ex-Lax	30–270-mg tabs
Antiemetics		
benzquinamide	Emete-Con	50 mg IM q3–4h PRN
prochlorperazine	Compazine	PO, IM, IV, or supp, 25 mg 5–10 mg PO or IM qid
trimethobenzamide	Tigan	PO, IM, or supp 250 mg tid or qid
promethazine	Phenergan	Tabs, syrup, IM, or supp 25 mg
dimenhydrinate	Dramamine	PO or IM 50–100 mg q4h PRN for motion sickness
scopolamine	Transderm-Scop, Scopolamine (injection)	0.5 mg q72h for motion sickness 0.3–0.6 mg preoperatively

Contraindications or extreme caution apply to:

Small children (increased risk of Reye's syndrome)
Pregnancy and lactation
Debilitated, emaciated, or geriatric patients
Angle-closure glaucoma
Prostatic hypertrophy

Interactions resulting in potentiation of a sedative effect occur with:

CNS depressants, including tranquilizers, hypnotics, and analgesics
Alcohol
Muscle relaxants

See Table 16.2 for a summary of laxatives and antiemetics.

PATIENT EDUCATION

Patients should be instructed regarding:

Taking these medications under medical supervision

Determining the cause of nausea and vomiting

Reporting effectiveness or complications

Administering only as directed

Not combining with any other CNS depressants, alcohol, or muscle relaxants unless prescribed by a physician (e.g., with cancer patients)

WORKSHEET FOR CHAPTER 16

Gastrointestinal Drugs

List the drugs according to category and complete all columns. Learn generic or trade names as specified by instructor.

CLASSIFICATIONS AND DRUGS	PURPOSE	SIDE EFFECTS	CONTRAINDICATIONS OR CAUTIONS	PATIENT EDUCATION
Antacids				
1.				
2.				
3.				
Antiulcer Agents				
1.				
2.				
Antidiarrhea Agents				
1.				
2.				
3.				
4.				
Antiflatulent				
1.				
Bulk-forming Laxative				
1.				

CLASSIFICATIONS AND DRUGS	PURPOSE	SIDE EFFECTS	CONTRAINDICATIONS OR CAUTIONS	PATIENT EDUCATION
Stool softeners				
1.				
2.				
Saline Laxative				
1.				
Stimulant Laxatives				
1.				
2.				
3.				
4.				
Antiemetics				
1.				
2.				
3.				
4.				
5.				
6.				

17

Antineoplastic Drugs

OBJECTIVES

Upon completion of this chapter, the student will be able to:

1. Define antineoplastic, chemotherapy, palliative, proliferation, cytotoxic, and immunosuppressive.
2. Name the six major groups of antineoplastic agents.
3. List the side effects common to most of the antineoplastic agents.
4. Describe appropriate interventions in caring for patients receiving antineoplastic agents.
5. Explain precautions in caring for those receiving radioactive isotopes.
6. Describe the responsibilities of those caring for patients receiving chemotherapy.
7. Explain appropriate education for patient and family when antineoplastic agents are administered.

Antineoplastic (against new tissue formation) refers to an agent that counteracts the development, growth, or spread of malignant cells. Cancer therapy frequently includes a combination of surgery, radiation, and/or chemotherapy.

Chemotherapy is a constantly growing field in which many old and new drugs and drug combinations are used for *palliative* effects (alleviation of symptoms), or for long-term or complete *remissions* in early treatment of cancer. Antineoplastic drugs are *cytotoxic* (destructive to cells), especially to cells that are proliferating (reproducing rapidly). Unfortunately, the toxic effects of the antineoplastic drugs are not confined to malignant cells alone, but also affect other proliferating) tissue, such as bone marrow, gastrointestinal epithelium, skin, hair follicles, and epithelium of the gonads, resulting in numerous adverse side effects.

Many antineoplastic agents also possess *immunosuppressive* properties, which decrease the production of antibodies and phagocytes, and reduce the inflammatory reaction. Suppression of the immune response results in increased susceptibility of the patient to infection.

Antineoplastic drugs are frequently administered in high doses on an *intermittent* schedule. Because most normal tissues have a greater capacity for repair than do most malignant tissues, normal cells may recover during the drug-free period.

Chemotherapy is *individualized* and frequently modified according to the patient's response to treatment. A *combination of several drugs* is frequently prescribed, with the choice of agents based on the type of malignancy, areas involved, extent of the cancer, physical condition of the patient, and other factors. Careful planning is required to maximize the effectiveness of therapy and to minimize the side effects and discomfort for the patient. Understanding of the treatment program and possible side effects is essential for all concerned: the nurse, the patient, and the family. Preplanning includes provision for symptomatic relief, such as antiemetics, as well as reassurance and availability of support staff to answer questions, explore feelings, and allay fears. Knowledge of side effects and appropriate interventions and patient education are essential for health care workers in this area.

Antineoplastic agents can be generally classified into six major groups: antimetabolites, alkylating agents, plant alkaloids, antitumor antibiotics, steroid hormones, and radioactive isotopes.

Antimetabolites

Antimetabolites are used in the treatment of leukemia, osteogenic sarcoma, squamous cell carcinoma, breast cancer, and other malignancies, especially those involving the genital areas. Some antimetabolites include methotrexate, fluorouracil, cytarabine, and 6-mercaptopurine. Methotrexate has also been used for severe, resistant cases of psoriasis.

Side effects can include:

Anorexia, nausea, vomiting, and diarrhea
Ulceration and bleeding of the oral mucosa and GI tract

Bone marrow depression, including leukopenia (infection), anemia and thrombocytopenia with hemorrhage

Rash, itching, photosensitivity, and scaling

Alopecia (regrowth of hair may take several months)

Contraindications or extreme caution applies to:

Renal and hepatic disorders
Pregnancy
GI ulcers

Alkylating Agents

Alkylating agents are used in the treatment of a wide range of cancers, including sarcomas, lymphomas, and leukemias. Some alkylating agents include carmustine, cisplatin, and thiotepa, used for metastatic ovarian, testicular, and bladder cancer and sometimes in palliative treatment of other cancers.

Side effects can include:

Nausea, vomiting, and diarrhea
Bone marrow depression, including leukopenia, with infection, anemia and thrombocytopenia with hemorrhage
Neurotoxicity, including headache, vertigo, and convulsions
Rash and alopecia
Loss of reproductive capacity

Contraindications or extreme caution applies to:

Debilitated patients
Pregnancy

Plant Alkaloids

Plant alkaloids are used in combination with other chemotherapeutic agents in the treatment of leukemias, Hodgkin's disease, lymphomas, sarcomas, and other malignancies. Some plant alkaloids include vinblastine and vincristine.

Side effects can include:

Neurotoxicity, including numbness; tingling; ataxia; foot drop; pain in jaw, head, or extremities; and visual disturbances
Severe constipation or diarrhea, nausea, and vomiting

Oral or GI ulceration

Rash, phototoxicity, and alopecia

Leukopenia with vinblastine (hematologic effects rare with vincristine)

Necrosis of tissue if infiltrated

Contraindications or caution applies to pregnancy.

Antitumor Antibiotics

Antitumor antibiotics are used to treat a wide variety of malignancies, including sarcomas, Hodgkin's disease, lymphomas, and tumors of the head and testicles. Antitumor antibiotics include bleomycin, dactinomycin, mitomycin, and others.

Side effects can include:

Nausea, vomiting, and diarrhea

Bone marrow depression

Cardiotoxicity, including arrhythmias and congestive heart failure

Pneumonitis, dyspnea and rales

Ulceration of mouth or colon

Alopecia, rash, and scaling

Contraindications or caution applies to:

Pregnancy

Liver disorders

Steroid Hormones

Corticosteroids, such as prednisone, are frequently used in combination with other chemotherapeutic agents in the treatment of leukemias and lymphomas. In addition, large doses of dexamethasone (Decadron) have been found effective in the prevention and treatment of nausea and vomiting associated with many neoplastic agents, when administered before or with chemotherapy.

Side effects with prolonged use of prednisone (see Chapter 23) include:

Fluid retention

Cushingoid features (moon face)

Fatigue and weakness

Osteoporosis

Sex hormones, including the estrogens, progestins, and androgens, are also used as antineoplastic agents in the treatment of malignancies involving the reproductive system (e.g., cancer of the breast, uterus, or prostate). These hormones are discussed in Chapter 24.

Radioactive Isotopes

Radioactive isotopes are also used in the treatment of certain types of cancer. Sometimes the radioactive material is injected into the affected site (e.g., radiogold, injected into the pleural or peritoneal cavity to treat ascites caused by cancer). Radioactive sodium iodine is administered PO or IV to treat thyroid cancer. Radioactive material is sometimes implanted in the body in the form of capsules, needles, or seeds.

Health care workers caring for patients receiving radioactive isotopes must observe special precautions to prevent unnecessary radiation exposure. Gowns and gloves should be worn when handling secretions. Other isolation procedures, such as handling of linens, will be outlined in the hospital procedure manual. This protocol should be followed with great care by all those who come in contact with patients receiving radioactive materials, for the protection of patients, as well as the health care worker.

Cautions for Antineoplastic Drugs

Health care workers involved in the administration of antineoplastic agents, as well as all those who care for these patients, have a number of very important responsibilities:

1. All medications should be given on time and exactly as prescribed to keep the patient as comfortable as possible.
2. Intravenous sites must be checked with great care because antineoplastic agents can cause extreme tissue damage and necrosis if infiltration occurs.
3. Intravenous fluids containing antineoplastic agents should not be allowed to get on the skin or into the eyes of the patient or the one administering the medication.
4. Antiemetics should be immediately available and administered as prescribed to minimize nausea and vomiting.
5. Careful and frequent oral hygiene is essential to minimize the discomfort and ulceration.
6. Soft foods and cool liquids should be available to the patient as required.

7. Accurate intake and output is important for adequate assessment of hydration.
8. Careful observation and reporting of symptoms and side effects is an essential part of chemotherapy.
9. Aseptic technique is necessary to minimize the chance of infection in patients with reduced resistance to infection.
10. Careful assessment of vital signs is important to identify signs of infection, cardiac irregularities, and dyspnea.
11. The health care worker must be informed about all aspects of chemotherapy and answer the patient's questions honestly. Awareness of verbal and nonverbal communication that gives clues to the patient's needs is absolutely necessary.
12. Careful attention to detail, astute observations, appropriate interventions, and compassion are an integral part of care when the patient is receiving chemotherapy.
13. The health care worker should reassure the patient that someone will be available to help at all times. Identify these resources.

PATIENT EDUCATION

Patients and their families should be instructed regarding:

Side effects to expect, how long they can be expected to continue, and that they are temporary

Comfort measures for coping with unpleasant side effects, (e.g., antiemetics as prescribed)

Appropriate diet with foods that are more palatable and more likely to be tolerated (e.g., soft foods, bland foods, a variety of liquids, and especially cold foods in frequent, small quantities)

Careful aseptic technique to decrease the chance of infections and reporting any signs of infection (e.g., fever)

Careful oral hygiene with swabs to prevent further trauma to ulcerated mucosa

Observation for bleeding in stools, urine, and gums and for bruises, and reporting this to medical personnel

Reporting of any persistent or unusual side effects, such as dizziness, severe headache, numbness, tingling, difficulty walking, or visaul disturbances

Available community resources to assist and support the patient (e.g., Cancer Society, Hospice, or Home Health services) as required and recommended by the physician

How to obtain information and answers to questions regarding treatment

The right of patients to terminate therapy if they wish

See Table 17.1 for a summary of the antineoplastic agents.

TABLE 17.1. ANTINEOPLASTIC AGENTS

Generic Name	Trade Name
Antimetabolites	
cytarabine	Cytosar-U
fluorouracil	5 FU
methotrexate	Mexate
6-mercaptopurine	Purinethol
Alkylating Agents	
carmustine	BCNU
cisplatin	Platinol
cyclophosphamide	Cytoxan
mechlorethamine	Mustargen
thiotepa	Thiotepa
Plant Alkaloids	
vinblastine	Velban
vincristine	Oncovin
Antitumor Antibiotics	
bleomycin	Blenoxane
dactinomycin	Actinomycin, Cosmogen
doxorubicin	Adriamycin
mitomycin	Mutamycin
Steroid Hormones	
dexamethasone	Decadron
prednisone	Deltasone

Note: This listing is not complete but is representative of the most used drugs. Dosage is on an intermittent schedule and individualized.

WORKSHEET FOR CHAPTER 17

Antineoplastic Drugs

Note the drugs listed according to category and complete all columns. See note on Table 17.1 regarding names of drugs.

CLASSIFICATIONS AND DRUGS	PURPOSE	SIDE EFFECTS	CONTRAINDICATIONS OR CAUTIONS	PATIENT EDUCATION
Antimetabolites				
1. fluorouracil				
2. methotrexate				
3. cytarabine				
4. 6-mercaptopurine				
Alkylating Agents				
1. carmustine				
2. cisplatin				
3. thiotepa				
Plant Alkaloids				
1. vinblastine				
2. vincristine				
Antitumor Antibiotics				
1. bleomycin				
2. dactinomycin				
3. mitomycin				

CLASSIFICATIONS AND DRUGS	PURPOSE	SIDE EFFECTS	CONTRAINDICATIONS OR CAUTIONS	PATIENT EDUCATION
Steroid Hormones 1. dexamethasone 2. prednisone				
Radioactive Isotopes				

18

Autonomic Nervous System Drugs

OBJECTIVES

Upon completion of this chapter, the student will be able to:

1. Define sympathomimetic and parasympathomimetic.
2. Compare and contrast characteristics of the four categories of autonomic nervous system drugs.
3. List the most frequently used (key) drugs in each of the four categories and the purpose of administration.
4. Describe the possible side effects of each of the key drugs.
5. Explain interactions and contraindications of the key drugs.

The autonomic nervous system (ANS) can be thought of as being *automatic,* self-governing, or involuntary. That is to say, we have no control over the action of the autonomic nervous system. Chemical substances called *mediators* are released at the nerve endings to transmit the nerve impulses from nerve to nerve at the synapses or from nerve to muscle at the myoneural junctions.

The autonomic nervous system is divided into the *sympathetic* and the *parasympathetic* divisions. Drugs that affect the function of the autonomic nervous system are divided into four categories:

1. Adrenergics (sympathomimetics)
2. Adrenergic blockers (beta blockers)
3. Cholinergics (parasympathomimetics)
4. Cholinergic blockers (anticholinergics)

Adrenergics

The sympathetic nervous system can be thought of as the emergency system used to mobilize the body for quick response and action. Key words to illustrate this action are *fright, fight,* and *flight.* If someone is startled in a dark place by a sudden motion, the body automatically mobilizes the sympathetic nerves to prepare the body to handle the fright by flight or a fight. The blood pressure, pulse, and respiration increase. The peripheral blood vessels constrict, sending more blood inward to the vital organs and skeletal muscles and speeding up the heart action. The bronchioles dilate to allow for a greater oxygen supply. The pupils dilate.

The chemical substances (mediators) released at the sympathetic nerve endings are called catecholamines and include epinephrine (*adrenalin*), norepinephrine, dopamine, and isoproterenol. Drugs that mimic the action of the sympathetic nervous system are called *sympathomimetic* or adrenergic.

Actions include:

Cardiac stimulation
Increased blood flow to skeletal muscles
Peripheral vasoconstriction
Bronchodilation
Dilation of pupils (mydriatic action)

Uses include:

Restoring rhythm in cardiac arrest
Elevating blood pressure in shock of all kinds
Constricting capillaries (e.g., to relieve nosebleed or nasal congestion or combined with local anesthetics for minor surgery)

Dilating bronchioles in acute asthmatic attacks, bronchospasm, or anaphylactic reaction

Ophthalmic procedures (mydriatic agent)

Side effects may include:

Palpitations

Nervousness or tremor

Tachycardia

Cardiac arrhythmias

Anginal pain

Hypertension

Tissue necrosis (when applied to lacerations of periphery, e.g., nose, fingers, and toes)

Glycosuria

Headache and insomnia

Contraindications or extreme caution applies to:

Angina

Coronary insufficiency

Hypertension

Cardiac arrhythmias

Angle-closure glaucoma

Organic brain damage

Hyperthyroidism

TABLE 18.1. ADRENERGICS

Generic Name	Trade Name	Dosage	Comments
epinephrine	Adrenalin	0.1–0.5 ml 1 : 1,000 sol SC or IM[a] 0.1–0.25 ml 1 : 1,000 sol IV[a]	For bronchospasm, asthma, cardiac arrest, anaphylaxis
ephedrine	Ephedrine	25–50 mg IM or SC 12.5–50 mg PO bid or qid	To raise blood pressure Nasal decongestant or bronchodilator
dopamine	Intropin	2–5 µg/kg/min IV	To raise blood pressure, cardiotonic
isoproterenol	Isuprel	10–20 mg SL q6–8h or inhalations qid .02–.2 mg IV or IM	For asthma or bronchospasm For heartblock or ventricular arrhythmias
metaraminol	Aramine	.5–5 mg IV	To raise blood pressure in shock
norepinephrine	Levophed	2–12 µg/min IV	For severe shock

[a]Use caution with dosage. This caution applies to both dosages.

Interactions may occur with:

CNS drugs (e.g., alcohol and antidepressants)
Propranolol (Inderal) or other beta-adrenergic blockers

See Table 18.1 for a summary of the adrenergics.

Adrenergic Blockers

Drugs that block the action of the sympathetic nervous system are called adrenergic blockers. The most commonly used drugs in this category are beta-adrenergic blockers, or *beta blockers*, such as propranolol (Inderal).

Uses of the beta blockers include:

Hypertension
Cardiac arrhythmias
Angina pectoris
Migraine headache

Side effects may include:

Hypotension
Bradycardia
Fatigue or lethargy
Nausea and vomiting
Hypoglycemia
Confusion

TABLE 18.2. ADRENERGIC BLOCKERS

Generic Name	Trade Name	Dosage	Comments
propranolol[a]	Inderal	PO 160–480 mg qd bid or tid	Begin with smaller dose and increase gradually to optimum dose for blood pressure control
		PO 10–20 mg qid	For angina
		PO 10–30 mg qid IV 1–5 mg *slowly*	For arrhythmias *extreme caution*
		PO 80-mg initial dose, increase to 160–240 mg qd	For migraine

[a]A beta-adrenergic blocker, or beta blocker.

Contraindications or extreme caution applies to:

Congestive heart failure of atrioventricular block
Hypotension
Asthma
Diabetes

Interactions may occur with:

Digitalis
Insulin or oral hypoglycemics
Aminophyllin
Isuprel
Epinephrine
Alcohol

PATIENT EDUCATION

Patients taking beta blockers, frequently given for cardiovascular disease, should be instructed regarding:

Rising slowly from reclining position to avoid postural hypotension
Possible slow heartbeat and reporting dizziness or excessive weakness to the physician
Avoiding alcohol, antihistamines, muscle relaxants, tranquilizers, and sedatives because they potentiate CNS depression and sedation
Reporting sexual dysfunction or depression to the physician for possible dosage regulation

---

Cholinergics

The parasympathetic nerve fibers synthesize and liberate *acetylcholine* as the mediator. Drugs that mimic the action of the parasympathetic nervous system are called *parasympathomimetic* or cholinergic drugs (e.g., bethanecol, neostigmine, and pilocarpine).

Actions include:

Increased gastrointestinal peristalsis
Increased contraction of the urinary bladder
Increased secretions (sweat, saliva, and gastric juices)
Increased skeletal muscle strength
Lowered intraocular pressure
Constriction of pupils
Slowing of the heart

Uses include treatment of:

Nonobstructive urinary retention (bethanecol)
Abdominal distention (neostigmine)
Myasthenia gravis (neostigmine)
Open-angle glaucoma (pilocarpine)
Pediculosis or as an insecticide (malathion)

Side effects may include:

Nausea, vomiting, and diarrhea
Muscle cramps and weakness
Slowing of the heart, hypotension, and bronchospasm
Sweating, excessive salivation, and lacrimation
Respiratory depression

Acute toxicity or cholinergic crisis is treated with atropine sulfate IV.

Contraindications or extreme caution applies to:

Benign prostatic hypertrophy (BPH)
Gastrointestinal disorders (e.g., ulcer and obstruction)
Asthma
Cardiac disorders

Interactions occur with:

Procainamide
Quinidine

See Table 18.3 for a summary of the cholinergics.

TABLE 18.3. CHOLINERGICS

Generic Name	Trade Name	Dosage	Comments
bethanecol	Urecholine	10–30 mg PO tid or qid	For urinary retention or abdominal distention, *not* with benign prostatic hypertrophy
edrophonium	Tensilon	1–2 mg IV, then 8 mg if no response	Test for myasthenia gravis
neostigmine	Prostigmin	15–375 mg PO in divided doses qd .5–2 mg IM or IV q1–3h.	Treatment for myasthenia gravis
pilocarpine	Isopto Carpine	Ophthalmic gtts, dose varies	To lower intraocular pressure with glaucoma

---

PATIENT EDUCATION

Patients taking cholinergic drugs or exposed to insecticides containing cholinergic agents (e.g., malathion) should be instructed regarding:

Reporting immediately to physician or emergency room any symptoms of prolonged GI distress (e.g., nausea, vomiting, and diarrhea), excessive perspiration, slow heartbeat, or depressed respiration

Avoiding combination of cholinergic medicatioins with heart medications or antibiotics

---

Cholinergic Blockers

Cholinergic blockers, or anticholinergics, are drugs that block the action of the parasympathetic nervous system. Atropine is the classic example of a cholinergic blocker. Others are listed in Table 18.4.

Actions include:

Drying (all secretions decreased)
Decreased GI and genitourinary (GU) motility
Dilation of pupils

Uses of atropine:

Antispasmodic and antisecretory for GI or GU hypermobility
Preoperative and preanesthetic uses
Drug-induced parkinsonism
Neuromuscular block and other spastic disorders

TABLE 18.4. CHOLINERGIC BLOCKERS

Generic Name	Trade Name	Dosage[b]	Comments
atropine	Atropine[b]	0.4–0.6 mg IM	Preoperative
		2 mg IM or IV qh	For insectide poisoning
		0.6–1 mg IV	For bradycardia or atrioventricular block
glycophyrrolate	Robinul	0.2 mg IM or IV	Preoperative
methanelamine	Banthine	50–100 mg PO qid	For ulcers, colitis, bladder spasm
	Pro-Banthine	15 mg PO qid	For ulcers, colitis
dicyclomine	Bentyl	10–20 mg PO qid	For ulcers, colitis
scopolamine		0.4–0.6 SC, patch	preoperative, antiemetic
homatropine[a]	Isopto Homatropine	Ophthalmic gtts	Mydriatic

[a]Other anticholinergics used in ophthalmic medications are discussed in Chapter 14.
[b]Use caution to give correct dosage.

Antidote for insecticide poisoning or cholinergic crisis

Emergency treatment of bradycardia and atrioventricular heart block with hypotension

Dilation of pupils (mydriatic)

Prevention and treatment of bronchospasm (bronchodilator)

Side effects of atropine may include:

Fever or flushing

Blurred vision

Dry mouth, constipation, and urinary retention

Confusion and headache

Palpitations and tachycardia

Contraindications or extreme caution applies to:

Asthma and other chronic pulmonary disease

Angle-closure glaucoma

GI or GU obstruction

Cardiac arrhythmias

Hypertension

Interactions with potentiation of sedation and drying occur with antihistamines (e.g., diphenhydramine).

PATIENT EDUCATION

Patients receiving cholinergic blockers should be instructed regarding:

Dried secretions (e.g., dry mouth)

Possible blurring of vision

Reporting fast heartbeat or palpitations

Avoiding anticholinergics with chronic obstructive lung disease and asthma

---

See Table 18.4 for a summary of the anticholinergics.

See Figure 18.1 for a summary of the autonomic nervous system drugs.

THE AUTONOMIC NERVOUS SYSTEM

| **Sympathetic** | **Parasympathetic** |

A = (Adrenergic) action

fright 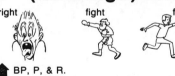 fight   flight

⬆ BP, P, & R.

FAST

bronchioles dilate
pupils dilate

peripheral blood vessels constrict

Adrenergic Drugs:

epinephrine (Adrenalin)
isoproterenol (Isuprel)
norepinephrine (Levophed)

side effects: tachycardia, palpitations, hypertension,
nervousness, glycosuria

C = (Cholinergic) action

⬆ secretions = fluids flow
⬆ peristalsis & bladder contractions
⬆ increased muscle strength
⬇ resp. slow & ⬇

 SLOW

 pupils constrict ⬇ intraocular pressure

Cholinergic Drugs:

bethenecol (Urecholine)
neostigmine (Prostigmine)
pilocarpine ophth. gtts

side effects: nausea, vomiting, diarrhea,
sweating, bradycardia, resp. ⬇

B = β-adrenergic Blockers

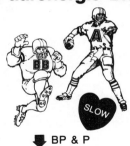

SLOW

⬇ BP & P

Beta blocker:

propranolol (Inderal)

side effects: hypotension, bradycardia,
fatigue, depression, hypoglycemia

D = Cholinergic Blockers

(3D effects)

drying
decreased motility G.I. & G.U.
dilated pupils

FAST

⬆ heart rate

Anticholinergic:

atropine

side effects: dry mouth, urinary retention,
constipation, blurred vision
confusion, tachycardia

Figure 18.1 *The autonomic nervous system drugs can be as simple as A, B, C, D.*

WORKSHEET FOR CHAPTER 18

Autonomic Nervous System Drugs

List the drugs according to category and complete all columns. Learn generic or trade names as specified by instructor.

CLASSIFICATIONS AND DRUGS	PURPOSE	SIDE EFFECTS	CONTRAINDICATIONS OR CAUTIONS	PATIENT EDUCATION
Adrenergics				
1.				
2.				
3.				
4.				
5.				
Adrenergic Blocker				
1.				
Cholinergics				
1.				
2.				
Cholinergic Blockers				
1.				
2.				
3.				
4.				

19

Analgesics, Sedatives, and Hypnotics

OBJECTIVES

Upon completion of this chapter, the student will be able to:

1. Define analgesic, sedative, hypnotic, subjective, objective, placebo, endorphin, narcotic, antipyretic, tinnitus, paradoxical, REM, and tolerance.

2. Compare and contrast the purpose and action of narcotic and nonnarcotic analgesics, sedatives, and hypnotics.

3. List the side effects of the major analgesics, sedatives, and hypnotics.

4. Describe the necessary information for patient education regarding interactions and cautions.

5. Explain the contraindications to administration of the CNS depressants in this chapter.

Analgesics, sedatives, and hypnotics depress central nervous system action to varying degrees. Some drugs can be classified in more than one category, depending on the dosage.

Analgesics are given for the purpose of relieving pain.
Sedatives are given to calm, soothe, or produce sedation.
Hypnotics are given to produce sleep.

Analgesics

Pain is subjective (i.e., it can be experienced or perceived only by the individual subject). Health care workers can view the patient's pain only in an objective way (i.e., observing the patient's reaction to pain in terms of vital signs, position, and emotional response). Pain has both psychological and physiological components. Some persons have a higher pain threshold than others because of conditioning, ethnic background, sensitivity, or physiological factors (e.g., endorphin release).

Endorphins are endogenous analgesics (produced within the body) as a reaction to severe pain or intense exercise (e.g., "runner's high"). Endorphin release may be responsible for a placebo effect: relief from pain as the result of suggestion without the administration of an analgesic.

NARCOTIC ANALGESICS

Analgesics can be classified as narcotic and nonnarcotic. Narcotics are sometimes called opiates, since the action is similar to that of opium in altering the perception of pain and in the potential for causing physical and psychological dependence. Narcotics are listed under the controlled substance schedule and include both the natural opium alkaloids (morphine and codeine) and the synthetics (e.g., Demerol and Darvon). Narcotics tend to cause *tolerance* with extended use (i.e., progressive decrease in effectiveness of the drug, with larger doses required to achieve the same effect). Because of tolerance, the potential for developing dependence, and the potentially serious CNS side effects, narcotics are not used for extended periods of time except to relieve chronic pain in terminal illness.

Side effects can include:

Sedation
Confusion, euphoria, restlessness, and agitation
Headache and dizziness
Hypotension and bradycardia
Nausea, vomiting, and constipation
Urinary retention
Respiratory depression
Physical and/or emotional dependence

Blurred vision
Convulsions with large doses
Flushing and rash

Contraindications or extreme caution applies to:

Head injury
CNS depression
Hepatic and renal disease
Hypothyroidism
COPD
Pregnancy, lactation, and pediatrics
Elderly and debilitated
Addiction-prone, suicidal, and alcoholic

Interactions include potentiation of effect with all CNS depressants, including:

Psychotropics
Alcohol
Sedatives and hypnotics
Muscle relaxants
Antihistamines
Antiemetics
Antiarrhythmics or antihypertensives
Frequently combined with phenergan postoperatively to potentiate analgesic effect

See Table 19.1 for a summary of the narcotic analgesics.

Narcotic antagonists are used in the treatment of narcotic overdoses and in the delivery room and newborn nursery for narcotic-induced respiratory depression. Two narcotic antagonists are nalorphine and naloxone:

Generic Name	Trade Name	Dosage
nalorphine	Nalline	1–4 mg IV, SC, or IM
naloxone	Narcan	may repeat q2–3min PRN × 3

NONNARCOTIC ANALGESICS

Nonnarcotic analgesics, many of which are available without prescription as over-the-counter medications, are very popular in this nation of "pill poppers." Therefore, it is extremely important that the health care worker be informed and responsible for patient education in this very important area of public health. The lay public needs to become aware of the dangers of self-medication, overdosage, side effects, and interactions, as well as the grave danger of poisoning to children and the elderly by inappropriate use of these readily available drugs.

The nonnarcotic analgesics are given for the purpose of relieving pain or for their antipyretic (fever-reducing) properties. The *salicylates* are most commonly

TABLE 19.1. NARCOTIC ANALGESICS[a]

Generic Name	Trade Name	Dosage	Comments
butorphanol	Stadol	1–4 mg IM q3–4h PRN	Can cause sweating or rash
codeine	Codeine[b]	15–60 mg PO, SC, IM q4h PRN	For mild to moderate pain, antitussive
dihydrocodeine with aspirin	Synalgos	1 cap q4h PRN	
hydromorphone	Dilaudid	1–6 mg PO q4–6h PRN 2–4 mg IM, SC, IV q4–6h PRN; 3mg rectal supp	For moderate to severe pain
meperidine	Demerol	50–150 mg PO, IM, IV q3–4h PRN	For moderate to severe pain or preoperatively
methadone	Dolophine	2.5–10 mg PO, IM, SC q4–12h PRN; 15–120 mg PO qd	For severe pain and for narcotic withdrawal
fentanyl	Innovar	50–100 mg IM	30–60 min preoperatively
morphine sulfate	Morphine, MS	5–15 mg IM, SC, IV 30–60 mg PO q4h PRN	For severe pain

oxycodone
  with aspirin
  with acetaminophen
	Percodan
	Tylox, Percocet
		1–2 tabs or 5 ml liquid PO or rectal supp PRN q6h	For moderate to severe pain, usually combined with aspirin or acetaminophen and caffeine

pentazocine	Talwin	50–100 mg PO q3–4h PRN 30 mg IM, IV, SC q3h PRN	For moderate to severe pain
propoxyphene HCl propoxyphene with acetaminophen	Darvon, Darvocet-N	65–100 mg PO q4h PRN	For mild to moderate pain; suicide potential, especially combined with alcohol
Brompton's mixture[c]		Dose varies q3–4h *around the clock*	For severe chronic pain of terminal cancer to keep pain from developing with less sedation

[a]Watch closely for side effects and dependency.
[b]Each Empirin #2 tablet contains 5 gr aspirin plus codeine 15 mg (¼ gr); #3, codeine 30 mg (½ gr); and #4, codeine 60 mg (1 gr). Each Tylenol #2 tablet or capsule contains 300 mg acetaminophen plus #2, codeine 15 mg (¼ gr); #3, codeine 30 mg (½ gr); and #4, codeine 60 mg (1 gr).
[c]Combination with varying amounts of morphine or methadone, cocaine or amphetamine, antiemetic (phenothiazines), and alcohol.

used for their analgesic and antipyretic, as well as their anti-inflammatory action. *Acetaminophen* and *phenacetin* have only analgesic and antipyretic action but do not affect inflammation. These three types of analgesic-antipyretics are frequently prescribed as combination products with other drugs.

SALICYLATES

Salicylate analgesic and anti-inflammatory actions are associated principally with inhibition of prostaglandins. The salicylates, e.g., aspirin (ASA), are also discussed in Chapter 21.

Side effects, especially with prolonged use and/or high dosages, can include:

Prolonged bleeding time
Gastric distress, ulceration, and bleeding
Tinnitus and hearing loss
Hepatitis
Rash, frequent bruising, or gingivitis
Coma, respiratory depression, or anaphylaxis, which can result from hypersensitivity or overdosage, especially with children
GI symptoms, which can be minimized by administration with food, milk, or a large glass of water or by using aspirin buffered with antacids or in enteric-coated form
Poisoning. Keep out of reach of children (especially flavored children's aspirin)

Contraindications include:

GI ulcer and bleeding
Bleeding disorders and patients taking anticoagulants
Hodgkin's disease
Asthma (may cause bronchospasm)
Children with influenzalike illness (because of the danger of Reye's syndrome)

Interactions occur with:

Alcohol (may precipitate GI bleeding)
Anticoagulants (potentiation)
Ammonium chloride (potentiation)
Cimetidine (potentiation)
Corticosteroids (decrease salicylate effect)

ACETAMINOPHEN

Acetaminophen (Tylenol) is used extensively in the treatment of mild to moderate pain and fever. It has *no* effect on inflammation. However, acetaminophen has fewer adverse side effects than the salicylates (e.g., does not cause gastric irritation or precipitate bleeding). Therefore, it is sometimes used for only its analgesic properties in treating the chronic pain of arthritis so that the salicylate dosage may be reduced to safer levels with fewer side effects in these patients.

Side effects are rare, but large doses can cause:

Severe liver toxicity
Rash or urticaria

Caution must be used with alcohol ingestion because of potential liver damage.

PHENACETIN

Phenacetin is currently available only in a limited number of combination analgesic preparations. Its continued use has been questioned because phenacetin use has been associated with some cases of chronic nephritis.

Side effects can include:

Kidney disorders
Hemolytic anemia
Nausea and vomiting
Rash

Contraindications or extreme caution applies to patients with:

Anemia
Cardiac disorders
Pulmonary disease
Kidney and liver disorders

See Table 19.2 for a summary of the nonnarcotic analgesics and antipyretics.

Sedatives and Hypnotics

Sedatives and hypnotics are controlled substances used to promote sedation in smaller doses and to promote sleep in larger doses. In addition, phenobarbital is used prophylactically with febrile children who are seizure prone or in the treatment of seizure disorders, frequently combined with phenytoin. Pentobarbital is also used as a preanesthesia medication. Some of the psychotropic drugs are also used as sedative-hypnotics and are discussed in Chapter 20.

The sedative-hypnotics are classified as barbiturates and nonbarbiturates. None of these medications should be used for extended periods of time except under close medical supervision, as in the treatment of epilepsy, because of the potential for psychological and physical dependence. In addition, these medications depress the REM (rapid-eye-movement, or dream) phase of sleep, and withdrawal after prolonged use can result in a severe rebound effect with nightmares and hallucinations. The nonbarbiturates depress REM sleep to a lesser degree than the barbiturates.

BARBITURATES

Barbiturates have been implicated in many suicides and fatalities due to accidental overdoses, especially when combined with other CNS depressants or alcohol.

TABLE 19.2. NONNARCOTIC ANALGESICS AND ANTIPYRETICS

Generic Name	Trade Name	Dosage	Comments
acetylsalicyclic acid	Aspirin, ASA, Empirin, Ascriptin, Bufferin	5–10 gr PO or rectal supp q4h PRN; large doses for arthritis	Give with milk or food
acetaminophen	Tylenol, Datril, Tempra	325–650 mg PO or rectal supp q4h PRN	No anti-inflammatory action
combinations[a]			
ASA and caffeine	Anacin		
ASA and meprobamate plus ethoheptazine citrate	Equagesic		
ASA and acetaminophen and caffeine	Excedrin		
chlorzoxazone and acetaminophen	Parafon Forte		

[a]Representative sample.

The elderly may manifest paradoxical reactions to the barbiturates, such as hyperexcitability, confusion, or hallucinations. Because of slower metabolism and impaired circulation and memory, the elderly or debilitated patient is particularly susceptible to ill effects and overdose, and should be encouraged to use more natural methods of combating insomnia, such as exercise during the day, avoiding heavy meals near bedtime, warm milk, back rubs, soft music, and other calming influences.

Side effects of the barbiturates can include:

"Hangover effect" including lethargy, incoordination, depression, and headache
Nausea and vomiting
Rash
Angioedema
Confusion and delirium
Respiratory depression
Coma
Fatal overdoses

NONBARBITURATES

Nonbarbiturates have been proclaimed as safer and having less potential for abuse then the barbiturates. However, recent statistics indicate growing misuse of these drugs with potentially fatal results as well. Only short-term use of any hypnotic is recommended.

Older nonbarbiturate hypnotics include the bromides and chloral hydrate. Newer drugs in this category include the benzodiazepines (e.g., flurazepam).

Side effects of the bromides and chloral hydrate include:

Nausea and vomiting
Rash
Dizziness
Ataxia

Side effects of flurazepam are infrequent but can include:

Leukopenia with prolonged use
Daytime sedation, confusion, and headache

Contraindications for all the sedative-hypnotics include:

Prolonged use
Addiction-prone patients
Depressed and mentally unstable patients
Elderly and debilitated patients
Pregnancy and lactation

Caution must be used with respiratory, renal, or liver disorders and with children.

TABLE 19.3. SEDATIVES AND HYPNOTICS

Generic Name	Trade Name	Dosage	Comments
Barbiturates			
amobarbital	Amytal	65–200 mg PO or IM hs	
butabarbital	Butisol	50–100 mg PO hs	
pentobarbital	Nembutal	100–200 mg PO, IM or rectal, hs or preoperatively 100–150 mg IV	Given only in emergency; injected *very slowly* IV; watch for respiratory arrest
phenobarbital	Luminal	30–120 mg PO qd in divided doses 100–320 mg PO or IM hs	For sedation or epilepsy; For insomnia
		100–300 mg IV only in emergency	Injected *very slowly* IV; watch for respiratory arrest
Nonbarbiturates			
chloral hydrate	Noctec	500 mg to 1 g PO or rectal hs	
ethchlorvynol	Placidyl	500 mg to 1 g PO 100–200 mg PO bid	For insomnia For sedation
flurazepam	Dalmane	15–30 mg PO hs	
temazepam	Restoril	15–30 mg PO hs	

Interactions of all the sedative-hypnotics with the following drugs can be dangerous and potentially fatal:

Psychotropic drugs
Alcohol
Muscle relaxants
Antiemetics
Antihistamines
Analgesics

See Table 19.3 for a summary of the sedatives and hypnotics.

PATIENT EDUCATION

Patients taking analgesics, sedatives, or hypnotics should be instructed regarding:

Potential for physical and psychological dependence and tolerance with narcotics, sedatives, and hypnotics

Taking only limited doses for short periods of time, *except* to relieve pain in terminal illness (in terminal cases, analgesics should be given on a regular basis around the clock to prevent or control pain)

Caution with interactions; *not* taking any other medications, (except under close medical supervision), that potentiate CNS depression (e.g., psychotropics, *alcohol*, muscle relaxants, antihistamines, antiemetics, cardiac medications, and antihypertensives)

Serious potential side effects with prolonged use or overdose of narcotics, sedatives, and hypnotics (e.g., oversedation, dizziness, headache, confusion, agitation, nausea, constipation, urinary retention, and *potentially fatal* respiratory depression, bradycardia, or hypotension)

Tolerance effect with prolonged use, with increasingly larger doses required to achieve the same effect

Potential for overdose of sedatives or hypnotics and paradoxical reactions with the elderly (e.g., confusion, agitation, hallucinations, and hyperexcitability)

Withdrawal after prolonged use of sedatives and hypnotics possibly leading to rebound effects with nightmares and hallucinations

Mental alertness and physical coordination impairment causing accidents or falls

Caution regarding OTC analgesic combinations and checking ingredients on the label; being aware of possible side effects with those containing aspirin (e.g., gastric distress or bleeding)

WORKSHEET FOR CHAPTER 19

Analgesics, Sedatives, and Hypnotics

Note the drugs listed according to category and complete all columns. Learn generic or trade names as specified by instructor.

CLASSIFICATIONS AND DRUGS	PURPOSE	SIDE EFFECTS	CONTRAINDICATIONS OR CAUTIONS	PATIENT EDUCATION
Narcotics				
1. codeine				
2. Synalgos				
3. meperidine (Demerol)				
4. morphine				
5. oxycodone (Percodan)				
6. Talwin				
7. Darvon				
Narcotic Antagonist				
1. Narcan				
Nonnarcotic Analgesics and Antipyretics				
1. aspirin				
2. acetominophen (Tylenol)				
Sedative-Hypnotic Barbiturates				
1. pentobarbital (Nembutal)				
2. phenobarbital (Luminal)				

CLASSIFICATIONS AND DRUGS	PURPOSE	SIDE EFFECTS	CONTRAINDICATIONS OR CAUTIONS	PATIENT EDUCATION
Sedative-Hypnotic Nonbarbiturates				
1. chloral hydrate (Noctec)				
2. flurazepam (Dalmane)				

20

Psychotropic Medications, Alcohol, and Drug Abuse

OBJECTIVES

Upon completion of this chapter, the student will be able to:

1. Define psychotropic, tranquilizer, phenothiazine, tricyclic, tardive dyskinesia, ataxia, paradoxical effect, and bipolar disorders.
2. Categorize the most commonly used psychotropic medications according to the following four classifications: CNS stimulants, antidepressants, antianxiety medications, and antipsychotic medications.
3. List the purpose, action, side effects, interactions, and contraindications for psychotropic medications in common use.
4. Describe the physiological effects of prolonged alcohol use.
5. Explain treatment of acute and chronic alcoholism.
6. Compare and contrast drug addiction and habituation.
7. Describe the effects of the three most commonly used illegal drugs.

Psychotropic refers to any substance that acts on the mind. Psychotropic medications are drugs that can exert a therapeutic effect on a person's mental processes, emotions, or behavior. Drugs used for other purposes can have psychotropic effects. Examples of other medications that affect mental functioning are anesthetics, analgesics, sedatives, hypnotics, and antiemetics, which are discussed in other chapters.

Psychotropic medications can be classified according to the purpose for administration. The four classes are CNS stimulants, antidepressants, antianxiety medications and antipsychotic medications.

CNS Stimulants

CNS stimulant medications are given for the purpose of promoting central nervous system functioning. One drug in this category, caffeine and sodium benzoate, has been used to treat respiratory depression associated with overdosage of CNS depressant drugs, alcoholic stupor, or neonatal apnea.

Other CNS stimulant drugs include the amphetamines and methylphenidate (Ritalin), which are used to treat hyperkinetic syndrome or minimal brain dysfunction in children and for narcolepsy. Ritalin is also occasionally used in the treatment of senile apathy. The use of amphetamines to reduce appetite in the treatment of obesity is *not* recommended because tolerance develops rapidly and physical or psychic dependence may develop within a few weeks. These drugs have a high potential for abuse and should be used only under medical supervision for diagnosed medical disorders.

Side effects of the amphetamines and methylphenidate can include:

Nervousness, insomnia, and irritability
Tachycardia, palpitations, hypertension, hypotension, and cardiac arrhythmias
Dizziness, headache, and blurred vision
GI disturbances, including anorexia, nausea, and vomiting

Contraindications or caution applies to:

Treatment for obesity (never more than 2 weeks)
Patients with anxiety or agitation
History of drug dependence or alcoholism
Hyperthyroidism
Diabetes and renal disorders
Cardiovascular disorders
Glaucoma
Children under 6 years old and pregnancy

See Table 20.1 for a summary of the CNS stimulants.

TABLE 20.1. CENTRAL NERVOUS SYSTEM STIMULANTS

Generic Name	Trade Name	Dosage	Comments
caffeine and sodium benzoate		500 mg IM or IV	To increase respiration in alcoholic stupor or drug overdose
amphetamines	Desoxyn, Dexedrine	5 mg bid or tid	For narcolepsy
methylphenidate	Ritalin	5–10 mg tid	For narcolepsy, hyperkinesis, or senile apathy

Antidepressants

Antidepressant medications, sometimes called mood elevators, are used primarily to treat patients with various types of depression. The two categories in general use are the tricyclic antidepressants and the monamine oxidase (MAO) inhibitors.

TRICYCLICS

The tricyclics have delayed action, elevating the mood and increasing alertness after 10–20 days. They are frequently given at bedtime because of a mild tranquilizing effect. They are used more frequently than the MAO inhibitors because of milder and fewer side effects, except with the elderly.

Side effects of the tricyclics, such as imipramine (Tofranil) are anticholinergic in action and can include:

Dryness of the mouth
Dizziness
Drowsiness and sleep disorders
Blurred vision
Constipation and urinary retention
Postural hypotension, cardiac arrhythmias, and palpitation
Confusion, especially in the elderly

Contraindications or extreme caution applies to:

Cardiac, renal, and liver disorders
Elderly
Glaucoma

Interactions may occur with other CNS drugs and alcohol.

MAO INHIBITORS

The MAO inhibitors, such as phenelzine (Nardil), have potentially *very serious side effects* and cannot be given until 2 weeks after the tricyclics have been discontinued.

Side effects are adrenergic in action and can include:

Nervousness, agitation, and insomnia
Headache
Hypertension or hypertensive crisis (can be fatal)
Tachycardia, palpitation, and chest pain
Nausea, vomiting, and diarrhea
Blurred vision

Contraindications apply to patients with cardiac and liver disease.

Interactions of the MAO inhibitors with some drugs and foods can cause *hypertensive crisis*, manifested by severe headache, palpitation, sweating, chest pain, possible intracranial hemorrhage, and even death. Interactions may occur with:

Adrenergic drugs, diuretics, insulin, and levodopa
Tricyclics, resulting in seizures, fever, hypertension, and confusion
CNS depressants, resulting in circulatory collapse
Foods containing tryamine, tryptamine, or tryptophan, such as yogurt, sour cream, all cheeses, liver (especially chicken), pickled herring, figs, raisins, bananas, pineapple, avocados, broad beans (Chinese pea pods), meat tenderizers, and *alcoholic beverages* (especially red wine and beer), and all fermented or aged foods (e.g., corned beef, salami, and pepperoni)

TRAZADONE

A newer antidepressant drug, unrelated to the tricyclics or MAO inhibitors, is *trazadone*, which also helps in relieving anxiety.

Side effects with trazadone are fewer than with tricyclics & MAO inhibitors, mild to moderate, dose-related and usually decrease after the first few weeks of therapy. Drowsiness or dizziness are the main side effects in early treatment.

LITHIUM

Recurrent, cyclic major depressions and bipolar disorders (manic-depressive) are treated *long-term* with lithium salts. A maintenance dose is established by

TABLE 20.2. ANTIDEPRESSANTS

Generic Name	Trade Name	Dosage	Comments
Tricyclics[a]			
amitriptyline	Elavil	75–250 mg qd	All of these drugs interact with CNS drugs.
desipramine	Norpramin	75–100 mg qd	
doxepin	Sinequan	75–100 mg qd	
imipramine	Tofranil	75–300 mg qd	Also effective for enuresis.
nortriptyline	Aventyl	30–75 mg qd	
protriptyline	Vivactil	20–60 mg qd	
MAO Inhibitors			
isocarboxazid	Marplan	10–30 mg qd	All of these drugs interact with many foods and other drugs in serious reactions.
phenelzine	Nardil	15–75 mg qd	
tranylcypromine	Parnate	20–30 mg qd	
Other Antidepressants			
trazodone	Desyrel	150–600 mg qd	
lithium	Lithobid, Eskalith	Dosage varies	Adjusted to maintain serum levels of 1–1.5 in treatment of bipolar disorders or *cyclic* major depressions.

Note: All of these tricyclics have a delayed action and mild tranquilizing effect.

monitoring blood levels. Daily serum levels are checked initially and every few months thereafter to maintain a level of 1–1.5 mEq/L. Patients must be monitored and alerted for signs of toxicity.

Side effects can include:

GI distress (usual initially and resolves)
Cardiac arrhythmias and hypotension
Polyuria (dehydration may cause acute toxicity)
Tremors

Signs of lithium toxicity can include:

Drowsiness, confusion, blurred vision, and photophobia
Seizures, coma, and cardiovascular collapse

Caution must be used with:

Cardiovascular and kidney disorders
Elderly and debilitated patients

See Table 20.2 for a summary of the antidepressants.

Antianxiety Medications

Antianxiety medications (e.g., benzodiazepines) are sometimes referred to as anxiolytics or minor tranquilizers. They are useful for the *short-term* treatment of (1) anxiety disorders, (2) neurosis while making the patient amenable to psychotherapy, (3) some psychosomatic disorders and insomnia, and (4) nausea and vomiting. Benzodiazpines, such as Valium, are also used as muscle relaxants, anticonvulsants or preoperatively. Anxiolytics, when given in small doses, can reduce anxiety and promote relaxation without causing sedation. Larger doses are sometimes prescribed at bedtime for their sedative effect. Minor tranquilizers should *not* be taken for prolonged periods of time because *tolerance and psychological dependence* may develop. *Sudden withdrawal after prolonged use may result in seizures.*

Side effects may include:

Mental depression, hallucinations, and confusion
Drowsiness, lethargy, and headache
Ataxia, tremor, and extrapyramidal reactions
Rash and itching
Sensitivity to sunlight

Contraindications or extreme caution applies to:

Mental depression
Suicidal tendencies
Depressed vital signs
Pregnancy, lactation, and children
Liver and kidney dysfunction
Elderly and debilitated patients (paradoxical reactions may occur)
Persons operating machinery

TABLE 20.3. ANTIANXIETY MEDICATIONS

Generic Name	Trade Names	Dosage	Comments
alprazolam	Xanax	0.25–0.5 mg tid	
chlordiazepoxide	Librium	5–10 mg qid	Larger doses IV with severe anxiety
chlorazepate	Tranxene	15–60 mg qd 7.5–15 mg qd	For elderly patients who are agitated
diazepam	Valium	2–10 mg qid	Do not mix in syringe with other medications, also used as muscle relaxant or IV in status epilepticus
hydroxyzine	Atarax Vistaril	25–100 mg qid or IM 200–400 mg qid	Also preoperative medication or an antiemetic
lorazepam	Ativan	2–3 mg qid	
meprobamate	Equanil, Miltown	200–400 mg qid	
oxazepam	Serax	10–15 mg tid or qid	

Interactions with potentiation of effect may occur with:

CNS depressants (e.g., analgesics, anesthetics, sedative-hypnotics, other muscle relaxants, antihistamines, and alcohol)
Anticoagulants, corticosteroids, digitalis, and phenytoin

See Table 20.3 for a summary of antianxiety medications.

Antipsychotic Medications

Antipsychotic medications, such as haloperidol (Haldol), are sometimes called *neuroleptics*. They are useful in three major areas:

Relieving symptoms of psychoses or severe neuroses, including delusions, hallucinations, confusion, anxiety, and agitation
Relieving nausea and vomiting
Potentiation of analgesics

Many of the antipsychotics are classified chemically as phenothiazines, for example, chlorpromazine (Thorazine). Dosage can be regulated to modify disturbed behavior and relieve anxiety in many cases without profound impairment of consciousness. Antipsychotics, such as promethazine (Phenergan), are sometimes combined with other drugs for potentiation of sedative or antiemetic action.

Side effects may include:

Postural hypotension, tachycardia, and vertigo
Dry mouth, blurred vision, and fever
Jaundice, rash, and photosensitivity
Confusion, drowsiness, and restlessness
Constipation and urinary retention
Extrapyramidal reactions, such as parkinson-like symptoms and tardive dyskinesia (involuntary movements, such as tics), with prolonged use and/or high doses
Hypersensitivity reactions

Contraindication exists for patients with severe depression.

Interactions may include:

Potentiation with CNS depressants
Antagonism with anticonvulsants (seizure activity may increase)

See Table 20.4 for a summary of the antipsychotic medications.
See Figure 20.1 for a summary of Psychotropic Drugs.

TABLE 20.4. ANTIPSYCHOTIC MEDICATIONS

Generic Name	Trade Name	Dosage	Comments
chlorpromazine	Thorazine	200–500 mg qd	Primarily for severe anxiety; also for nausea and vomiting
haloperidol	Haldol	1–20 mg qd PO or IM	For agitation, especially with schizophrenia and confusion in the elderly
prochloperazine	Compazine	PO, supp, or IM	For agitation; primarily for nausea and vomiting
promethazine	Phenergan	12.5–25 mg qid, PO, supp, or IM	Primarily for nausea and vomiting pre- and postoperatively
thioridazine	Mellaril	10–100 mg qid	For psychoneurosis, agitation, or intractable pain
trifluoperazine	Stelazine	1 mg tab bid	Tranquilizer or antiemetic; low sedation
thiothixene	Navane	2–10 mg tid PO or IM	For chronic schizophrenic or behavioral management of retarded or Alzheimer's patients

There is no "ideal" psychotropic medication. All have side effects, and prolonged use can lead to addiction or habituation. However, research indicates a chemical component in many forms of mental illness. By altering abnormal levels of certain chemicals in the brain, such as dopamine or norepinephrine, many patients with mental or emotional illness have been helped. Psychiatric hospitalization has decreased since the advent of psychotropic medications.

Alcohol

Alcohol can be classified as a psychotropic drug and a CNS depressant. It is the number one drug problem in the United States.

Alcohol is a fast-acting depressant, pharmacologically similar to ether. The body reacts to both drugs with excitement, sedation, and finally anesthesia. Large amounts of alcohol can result in alcoholic stupor, cerebral edema, and depressed respiration.

Alcohol is rapidly absorbed from the GI tract into the bloodstream. Alcohol depresses primitive areas of the cortex first and then decreases control over judgment, memory, and other intellectual and emotional functioning. Within a few hours, motor areas are affected, producing unsteady gait, slurred speech, and incoordination. Prolonged use can cause permanent CNS damage and result in peripheral neuritis, convulsive disorders, Wernicke's syndrome, and Korsakoff's psychosis with mental deterioration, memory loss, and ataxia.

Prolonged alcohol use affects almost all organs of the body. Chronic drinking causes liver damage and pancreatitis. Alcohol irritates the mucosa of the digestive system, leading to possible esophageal varices, gastritis, ulceration, and hemorrhage. Alcohol can also lead to malabsorption of nutrients and malnutrition.

Cardiovascular effects include peripheral vasodilation (producing the flushing and sweating seen with intoxication) and vasoconstriction of the coronary arteries. Alcohol increases the heart rate and, with chronic use, can cause cardiac myopathy, either directly or through metabolic and electrolyte imbalances. Potassium deficiency can cause cardiac arrhythmias.

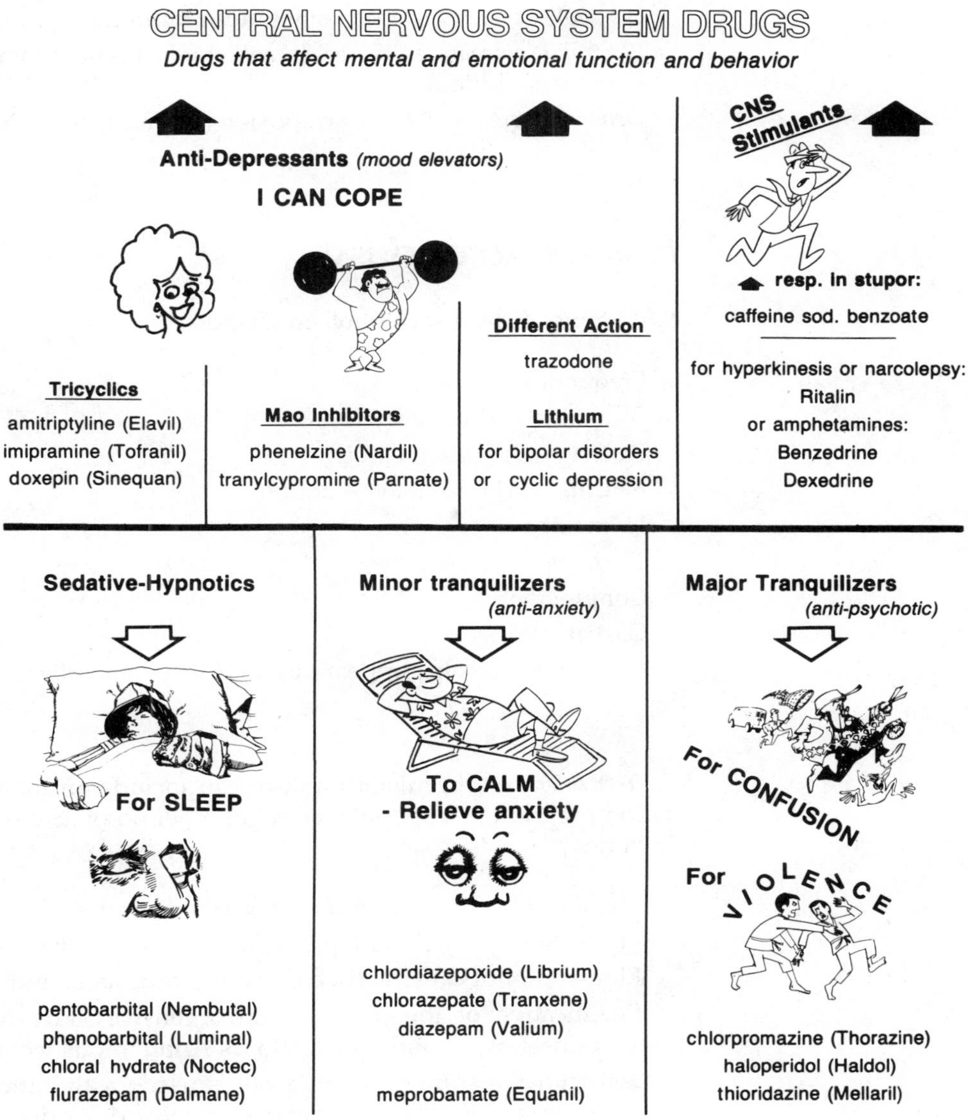

CENTRAL NERVOUS SYSTEM DRUGS

Drugs that affect mental and emotional function and behavior

Anti-Depressants *(mood elevators)*

I CAN COPE

Tricyclics

amitriptyline (Elavil)
imipramine (Tofranil)
doxepin (Sinequan)

Mao Inhibitors

phenelzine (Nardil)
tranylcypromine (Parnate)

Different Action

trazodone

Lithium

for bipolar disorders
or cyclic depression

CNS Stimulants

resp. in stupor:

caffeine sod. benzoate

for hyperkinesis or narcolepsy:
Ritalin
or amphetamines:
Benzedrine
Dexedrine

Sedative-Hypnotics

For SLEEP

pentobarbital (Nembutal)
phenobarbital (Luminal)
chloral hydrate (Noctec)
flurazepam (Dalmane)

Minor tranquilizers
(anti-anxiety)

**To CALM
- Relieve anxiety**

chlordiazepoxide (Librium)
chlorazepate (Tranxene)
diazepam (Valium)

meprobamate (Equanil)

Major Tranquilizers
(anti-psychotic)

For CONFUSION

For VIOLENCE

chlorpromazine (Thorazine)
haloperidol (Haldol)
thioridazine (Mellaril)

Figure 20.1 *Central nervous system drugs. Psychotropics.*

ALCOHOL POISONING

Symptoms of acute alcoholic poisoning include cold, clammy skin; stupor; slow, noisy respirations; and alcoholic breath.

Treatment includes close observation for:

Respiratory problems. Establish and maintain airway, give caffeine and sodium benzoate for depressed respirations.

Vomiting. Gastric lavage if indicated.

Convulsions. Phenytoin sometimes given prophylactically to decrease seizure activity.

Cerebral edema. Diuretics sometimes required (e.g., mannitol).

Electrolyte imbalance. IV fluids with high doses of vitamin B complex and vitamin C added.

Delirium tremens. Chlordiazepoxide (Librium) sometimes given.

CHRONIC ALCOHOLISM

Symptoms of chronic alcoholism include:

Frequent falls and accidents
Blackouts and memory loss
Dulling of mental faculties
Neuritis and muscular weakness
Irritability
Tremors
Conjunctivitis
Gastroenteritis
Neglect of personal appearance and responsibilities

Treatment of chronic alcoholism can include an intensive in-house rehabilitation program in a special facility for a period of 28 days. Treatment frequently includes:

Megadoses of vitamin B complex and vitamin C IM or PO
Low-carbohydrate and high-protein diet to combat hypoglycemia
Elimination of caffeine (in coffee, tea, chocolate, and soft drinks)
Reeducation of the patient, with intensive individual, group, and family counseling, including Alcoholics Anonymous techniques
Sometimes disulfiram (Antabuse) is used, with patient cooperation, as part of *behavior modification*. Patients receive daily doses of disulfiram and are taught to expect a very unpleasant reaction if even a small amount of alcohol is ingested.

Disulfiram-alcohol reactions can include:

Flushing and throbbing headache
Nausea and vomiting
Sweating and dyspnea
Palpitation, tachycardia, and hypotension
Vertigo and blurred vision
Anxiety and confusion

PATIENT EDUCATION

Patients taking disulfiram should be instructed regarding:

Avoidance of cough syrups, sauces, vinegars, elixirs, and other preparations containing alcohol

Caution with external applications of liniments, lotions, aftershave, or perfume

Signs of disulfiram-alcohol reaction

Reporting to emergency facility if effects do not subside or with severe reaction

Carrying identification card noting therapy

Avoiding other medications that may interact with disulfiram (e.g., anticoagulants and phenytoin)

Drug Abuse

Drug abuse can be defined as the use of a drug for other than therapeutic purposes. Drug *addiction* consists of the combination of all four of the following side effects: tolerance, psychological dependence, physical dependence, and withdrawal reaction with physiological effects. *Habituation* consists of psychological dependence only.

The sedative-hypnotic medications are the most frequently abused drugs, especially by medical personnel. Counteractive measures include accurate record keeping of all controlled substances, especially depressants and narcotics. Analgesics, sedatives, and hypnotics are discussed in Chapter 19 along with treatment for overdose and description of narcotic antagonists. This chapter describes only three types of illegal drugs: marijuana, cocaine, and the hallucinogens LSD and PCP.

MARIJUANA

Tetrahydrocannabinol (THC) is commonly known as marijuana. Although classified technically as a CNS depressant, it also possesses properties of a euphoriant, sedative, and hallucinogen. Marijuana is currently under investigation as a possible treatment for glaucoma and also for the vomiting associated with chemotherapy.

The *Cannabis* plant grows over the entire world, especially in tropical areas. Potency varies considerably from place to place and time to time. Marijuana is much more potent today than a few years ago.

THC, the active ingredient released when marijuana is smoked, is fat soluble and is stored in many fat cells, especially in the brain and reproductive organs. THC metabolizes slowly. A week after a person smokes one marijuana cigarette, 30%–50% of the THC remains in the body, and 4–6 weeks are required to eliminate all the THC.

Side effects include:

Short-term memory loss, impaired learning, and slowed intellectual performance
Perceptual inaccuracies (dangerous with driving)
Apathy, lethargy, and decreased motivation
Increased heart rate
Lung irritation and chronic cough
Reduced testosterone level and sperm count
Reduced estrogen level, crossing of placental barrier, and transmission through mother's milk
Delayed development of coping mechanisms in children and adolescents

COCAINE

Cocaine use is increasing in the United States. It is a CNS stimulant and produces euphoria and increased expenditure of energy. The only approved medical use is as a local anesthetic, usually for nasal procedures.

The drug abuser usually sniffs the white powder. This practice leads to the degeneration of the nasal septum. Sometimes cocaine is self-administered intravenously, a dangerous practice, occasionally fatal. Cocaine is also smoked. Used in this fashion, cocaine is rapidly addictive and extremely dangerous. Severe depression can be associated with withdrawal, which is a lengthy process.

Side effects include:

Euphoria, agitation, and excitation
Increased pulse and blood pressure
Anorexia, nausea, and GI disturbances
Hallucinations and possible psychosis
Convulsions
Possible death from circulatory collapse

HALLUCINOGENS

Lysergic acid (LSD) and phencyclidine (PCP), an animal tranquilizer, are hallucinogens. They produce bizarre mental reactions and distortion of physical senses. Hallucinations and delusions are common, with confused perceptions of time and space (e.g., the user can walk out of windows because of the impression that he or she can fly). PCP is also an amnesic.

Side effects of both include:

Increased pulse and heart rate and rise in blood pressure and temperature
Possible "flashbacks" months later
Panic or paranoia (lack of control)
Possible psychotic episodes
Possible physical injury to self or others

THE ROLE OF MEDICAL PERSONNEL

The role of medical personnel in combating drug abuse includes:

Thorough knowledge of psychotropic drugs, action, and side effects

Willingness to participate in education of the patient, the patient's family, and others in the community

Giving competent care to those under the influence of drugs in a nonjudgmental way

Recognizing drug abuse and making appropriate referrals

It is the responsibility of all medical personnel, not only to recognize drug abuse, but also to report any observed drug abuse to the *proper person in authority*. To look the other way not only enables the individual to continue to harm him- or herself, but also endangers those in his or her care.

PATIENT EDUCATION

Patients taking psychotropic drugs should be instructed regarding:

Potential for psychological and/or physical dependence with prolonged use

Caution in taking medication only in prescribed dosage and for limited period of time under medical supervision to reduce possibility of serious side effects from overdose or prolonged use

Reporting adverse side effects to physician at once (e.g., dizziness, blurred vision, nervousness, palpitations and other cardiac symptoms, urinary retention, GI symptoms, adverse mental changes, and extrapyramidal reactions)

Avoiding chemical abuse (e.g., alcohol or drugs) and obtaining professional treatment when these conditions exist

Possible severe withdrawal reactions (e.g., seizures) after prolonged use of psychotropic medications (withdrawal should never be abrupt, and medical supervision is indicated for prolonged administration of any of the psychotropic drugs)

Caution with interactions; *not* taking any other medications (except under close medical supervision) that can potentiate CNS depression (e.g., analgesics, *alcohol*, muscle relaxants, antihistamines, antiemetics, cardiac medications, or antihypertensives)

WORKSHEET 1 FOR CHAPTER 20

Psychotropics

Note the drugs listed according to category and complete all columns. Learn generic or trade names as specified by instructor. Fill in blank spaces in first column with names of other drugs common in your area.

CLASSIFICATIONS AND DRUGS	PURPOSE	SIDE EFFECTS	CONTRAINDICATIONS OR CAUTIONS	PATIENT EDUCATION
CNS Stimulants				
1. caffeine sodium benzoate				
2. amphetamines				
3. Ritalin				
Tricyclics				
1. Elavil				
2. Tofranil				
MAO Inhibitors				
1. Marplan				
2. Nardil				
Other Antidepressants				
1. lithium				

CLASSIFICATIONS AND DRUGS	PURPOSE	SIDE EFFECTS	CONTRAINDICATIONS OR CAUTIONS	PATIENT EDUCATION
Antianxiety Medications 1. Tranxene 2. Valium 3. meprobamate 4. 5.				
Antipsychotic Medications 1. Thorazine 2. Haldol 3. Mellaril 4. Navane 5.				
Illegal Drugs 1. marijuana 2. cocaine				

WORKSHEET 2 FOR CHAPTER 20

Alcohol

Complete the columns including medications and cautions under treatment. Learn generic or trade names as specified by instructor.

DIAGNOSIS	SIGNS AND SYMPTOMS	POSSIBLE EFFECTS ON THE BODY	TREATMENT
Chronic alcoholism			
Acute alcoholic poisoning			

21

Musculoskeletal and Anti-inflammatory Drugs

OBJECTIVES

Upon completion of this chapter, the student will be able to:

1. Identify commonly used skeletal muscle relaxants.
2. Describe the side effects to be expected with muscle relaxants.
3. List the drugs that can interact with the muscle relaxants and cause serious potentiation of effect.
4. Differentiate between the anti-inflammatory drugs, antirheumatic drugs, and drugs used to treat acute episodes of gout.
5. Explain the serious side effects of NSAID.
6. List drug interactions with NSAID.
7. Explain appropriate patient education for those taking skeletal muscle relaxants and NSAID.

Disorders of the musculoskeletal system are rather common. Drugs used to treat such conditions may be classified in two broad categories: skeletal muscle relaxants and nonsteroidal anti-inflammatory drugs (NSAID). Corticosteroid therapy for inflammatory conditions is discussed in Chapter 23.

Skeletal Muscle Relaxants

Some disorders of the musculoskeletal system can be attributed to structural defects (e.g., ruptured disks) that may require surgical intervention rather than medication. However, many disorders associated with pain, spasm, abnormal contraction, or impaired mobility do respond to medications classified as skeletal muscle relaxants. Acute, painful musculoskeletal conditions, such as backache or neck strain, are treated with a combination of muscle relaxants, rest, physical therapy (e.g., hot packs), and mild analgesics (e.g., aspirin). Muscle relaxants are given only on a short-term basis, and, after the acute pain subsides, exercises are usually prescribed by the physician to strengthen the weak muscles.

Muscle relaxant drugs can affect the spinal cord and brain, as well as acting on the peripheral areas. The resulting action not only reduces muscle spasm but produces a sedative effect, promoting rest and relaxation of the affected part. Drugs used to treat acute, painful musculoskeletal conditions include diazepam (Valium) and methocarbamol (Robaxin). See Table 21.1 for others.

A different type of muscle relaxant, dantrolene, causes a direct effect on skeletal muscles and is used in the management of spasticity resulting from upper motor neuron disorders such as multiple sclerosis or cerebral palsy. This medication is ineffective for amyotropic lateral sclerosis and is *not* indicated for the treatment of muscle spasms resulting from rheumatic disorders or musculoskeletal trauma.

Another type of muscle relaxant includes neuromuscular blocking agents such as succinylcholine or tubocurarine, used during surgical, endoscopic, or orthopedic procedures. These drugs are potentially *very dangerous* and can result in respiratory arrest. Neuromuscular blocking agents are administered only by anesthesiologists or specially trained personnel skilled in intubation and cardiopulmonary resuscitation.

Muscle relaxants need to be used with caution because of possible serious CNS problems, such as respiratory arrest and allergic reactions. Antidotes may be indicated, such as neostigmine (Prostigmin) or edrophonium (Tensilon). Prostigmin may also be used in treatment of myasthenia gravis and Tensilon in the diagnosis of myasthenia gravis.

Side effects can include:

Drowsiness and dizziness
Weakness and tremor
Headache
Confusion and nervousness
Ataxia
Slurred speech

Blurred vision
Hypotension
GI symptoms, including nausea, vomiting, diarrhea, and constipation
Urinary problems, including enuresis, frequency, and retention
Allergic and anaphylactic reactions
Respiratory depression

Contraindications are:

Muscular dystrophy
Myasthenia gravis
Pregnancy or lactation
Children under 12 years old

Caution should be used with:

Impaired kidney function
Liver disorders
Blood dyscrasias
Asthma
Cardiac disorders

Interactions with possible potentiation effect, may occur with:

Alcohol
Analgesics
Psychotropic medications
Antihistamines

PATIENT EDUCATION

Patients taking skeletal muscle relaxants should be instructed regarding:

Potential side effects (e.g., drowsiness, dizziness, weakness, tremor, blurred vision, hypotension, respiratory distress, or GI disorders)

Avoidance of other CNS depressants at the same time (e.g., tranquilizers, antihistamines, or alcohol), which can cause serious CNS depression, and care with analgesics, only as prescribed by a physician

Importance of following the physician's orders regarding rest and physical therapy (e.g., heat and firm mattress or bed board with back problems) and exercises as prescribed, (after the acute pain subsides), to strengthen the weak muscles

Taking the medication only as long as absolutely necessary and observing caution regarding prolonged use, which could lead to physical or psychological dependence and withdrawal symptoms (e.g., seizures from Valium withdrawal after prolonged use)

See Table 21.1 for a summary of the skeletal muscle relaxants.

TABLE 21.1. SKELETAL MUSCLE RELAXANTS

Generic Name	Trade Name	Dosage	Comments
carisoprodol	Soma, Rela	350 mg PO qid	Caution with asthma.
cylobenzaprine	Flexeril	30–60 mg PO qid in divided doses	For acute painful musculoskeletal conditions.
diazepam	Valium	2–10 mg PO qid IM, IV 2–20 mg q3–4h	Abrupt withdrawal after prolonged use may cause seizures.
methocarbamol	Robaxin	4–8 g PO qd in divided doses; also IM, IV	For acute painful musculoskeletal conditions.
dantrolene	Dantrium	25–100 mg PO qid	For multiple sclerosis and cerebral palsy; *not* for trauma or rheumatic disorders.

Anti-inflammatory Drugs

Anti-inflammatory drugs are used to treat disorders in which the musculoskeletal system is not functioning properly due to inflammation. Such conditions as arthritis, bursitis, spondylitis, gout, and muscle strains and sprains can cause swelling, redness, heat, pain, and limited mobility. Analgesics and corticosteroids are used at times for acute stages of these disorders and are discussed in Chapters 19 and 23. The corticosteroids are *not* used for extended periods of time because of serious side effects. However, nonsteroidal anti-inflammatory drugs (NSAID) are frequently given for lengthy time periods in maintenance doses as low as possible for effectiveness.

NONSTEROIDAL ANTI-INFLAMMATORY DRUGS

NSAID inhibit synthesis of prostaglandins, substances responsible for producing much of the inflammation and pain of rheumatic conditions, sprains and menstrual cramps. *No cure* has been found for rheumatic disorders but many medications are used to alleviate the pain and crippling effects. Because of lower metabolic rates, and other complications, the elderly are particularly susceptible to side effects from NSAID and should be cautioned to report any untoward signs or symptoms to their doctor without delay. Periodic lab tests are required for those on maintenance doses of NSAID to monitor effects.

The salicylates are the oldest drug in this category with analgesic, anti-inflammatory and antipyretic effects. Although safer than many of the newer, more potent antirheumatic drugs, side effects are still frequent, especially in the high doses required for effectiveness.

Side effects frequently include:

GI ulceration and bleeding
Epigastric pain, nausea, and heartburn

Constipation

Tinnitus and hearing loss

Headache

Dizziness

Nervousness

Visual disturbances

Hematuria and albuminuria

Peripheral edema

Rash, hypersensitivity reactions

Blood dyscracias (especially phenylbutazone)

Contraindications or extreme caution applies to:

Cardiovascular disorders

Kidney disease

Liver dysfunction

GI ulcer

Blood dyscracias

Thyroid disease

Children with viral infections (danger of Reye's syndrome)

These medications should be given with meals or milk to reduce GI side effects. Enteric-coated, timed-release capsules or buffered aspirin are sometimes also recommended to reduce gastric irritation.

PATIENT EDUCATION

Patients should be instructed regarding:

Administration with food to reduce gastric irritation

Caution with dosage (follow physician's directions carefully regarding amount of drug to reduce chance of overdose)

Discontinuing drug and reporting to physician any sign of abnormal bleeding (gums, stool, urine, and bruising), epigastric pain or nausea, ringing in the ears or hearing loss, visual disturbances, weight gain or edema, and skin rash

Avoiding taking any other drugs, either prescribed or OTC, without checking first with a physician or pharmacist regarding possible interactions

When taking gout medications (e.g., colchicine), always taking large amounts of fluids

Avoiding taking large amounts of aspirin or other NSAID with kidney, liver, or heart disease or with history of GI ulcer (with these conditions, take only under medical supervision)

TABLE 21.2. NONSTEROIDAL ANTIINFLAMMATORY DRUGS AND GOUT MEDICATION

Generic Name	Trade Name	Dosage	Comments
ibuprofen	Motrin, Advil (OTC), Nuprin (OTC)	300–600 mg PO qid	Watch for prolonged bleeding time.
indomethacin	Indocin	Up to 200 mg qd PO divided doses	
mefenamicacid	Ponstel	250 mg q4h PRN	For dysmenorrhea.
naproxen	Naprosyn, Anaprox	250–500 mg PO bid	For pain and dysmenorrhea.
phenylbutazone	Butazolidin	100–200 mg PO qid	For arthritis, bursitis, and acute gouty arthritis.
piroxicam	Feldene	20 mg PO qd	Watch for prolonged bleeding time.
sulindac	Clinoril	150–200 mg PO bid	For arthritis, spondylitis, and dysmenorrhea.
Gout medication colchicine	Colchicine	0.5–1.8 mg PO qd	Preventive or treatment for acute attacks of gout.

Interactions (especially of salicylates) are many, but the most important clinically occur with:

Alcohol, which potentiates possibility of GI bleeding
Anticoagulants, which potentiate possibility of bleeding
Sulfonylureas (oral hypoglycemics), which potentiate hypoglycemia
Corticosteroids, which potentiate salicylate absorption
Methotrexate, with potentiation and increased risk of methotrexate toxicity
Uricosurics (Benemid or Anturane), whose action is antagonized by salicylates

See Table 21.2 for a summary of the nonsteroidal anti-inflammatory drugs.

GOUT MEDICATIONS

Gout is a metabolic disorder characterized by accumulation of uric acid crystals in various joints, especially the big toe, ankle, knee, and elbow, with resultant pain and swelling. Colchicine is a specific drug that is used to relieve inflammation in *acute* gouty arthritis. It is also used as a prophylaxis in persons prone to this condition.

Side effects can include:

Rash
GI upset
Blood disorders

Always encourage large fluid intake to facilitate excretion of uric acid crystals. Other medications for *chronic* gout are discussed in Chapter 15. They act in a different way and are *not* effective against inflammation in acute cases of gout or gouty arthritis.

WORKSHEET FOR CHAPTER 21

Musculoskeletal and Anti-inflammatory Drugs

Note the drugs listed and complete all columns. Learn generic or trade names as specified by instructor.

CLASSIFICATIONS AND DRUGS	PURPOSE	SIDE EFFECTS	CONTRAINDICATIONS OR CAUTIONS	PATIENT EDUCATION
Skeletal Muscle Relaxants				
1. Flexeril				
2. Valium				
3. Robaxin				
4. Soma				
NSAID				
1. ibuprofen OTC				
2. Indocin				
3. Naprosyn				
4. Butazolidin				
Gout Medication (Anti-inflammatory)				
1.				

22

Anticonvulsants and Antiparkinsonian Drugs

OBJECTIVES

Upon completion of this chapter, the student will be able to:

1. Compare and contrast three different types of seizures: grand mal, petit mal, and psychomotor.
2. List the medications used for each type of epilepsy and common side effects.
3. List the drugs used for parkinsonism and common side effects.
4. Describe the patient education appropriate for those receiving anticonvulsants and antiparkinsonian drugs.

Anticonvulsants

Anticonvulsants are used to reduce the number and/or severity of seizures in patients with epilepsy. Epilepsy is defined as a *recurrent* paroxysmal disorder of brain function characterized by sudden attacks of altered consciousness, motor activity, or sensory impairment. Seizures may be classified as grand mal, psychomotor, or petit mal. Treatment is based on type, severity, and cause of seizures.

GRAND MAL AND PSYCHOMOTOR SEIZURES

Grand mal seizures are characterized by loss of consciousness, falling, and tonic followed by clonic contractions of the muscles. The attack is *generalized* and usually lasts 2–5 min. Initial treatment consists *only* in preventing injury by removing any objects that could cause trauma, cushioning the head and turning it to the side, and loosening tight clothing, especially collars and belts. Do *not* try to open the mouth or force anything between the teeth.

If seizures are so frequent that the patient does not regain consciousness between seizures, the condition is known as *status epilepticus*. The treatment of choice is IV diazepam (Valium) administered slowly.

Psychomotor epilepsy is caused by a lesion in the *temporal lobe* of the brain. It is characterized by momentary loss of consciousness, confusion, loss of judgment, and abnormal acts, even crimes and hallucinations, but no convulsions.

Prophylactic treatment of grand mal and psychomotor epilepsy usually consists of phenytoin (Dilantin), frequently combined with phenobarbital, administered orally. The aim of therapy is to prevent seizures without oversedation, and the dosage will be adjusted according to the individual patient's response.

Side effects of phenytoin (Dilantin), which frequently decrease with continued treatment, can include:

Sedation, ataxia, dizziness, and headache
Blurred vision, nystagnus, and diplopia
Gingivitis (inflamed gums)
GI distress, including nausea, vomiting, anorexia, constipation, and diarrhea
Rash and dermatitis (discontinue medication)
Megaloblastic anemia (treated with folic acid)
Osteomalacia (bone softening, treated with vitamin D)

Contraindications or extreme caution applies to:

Kidney or liver disease
Diabetes
Congestive heart failure, bradycardia, heart block, and hypotension
Pregnancy and lactation

An alternative medication in treatment of grand mal and psychomotor epilepsy is primidone (Mysoline), which has fewer side effects than phenytoin.

Febrile convulsions in children are frequently treated with phenobarbital alone.

PETIT MAL SEIZURES

Petit mal, or absence, epilepsy is so called because of the absence of convulsions. It is characterized by a 10–30-sec loss of consciousness with no falling. Partial seizure disorder is another term for this condition.

The drug of choice for management of petit mal epilepsy is ethosuximide (Zarontin), which is effective only for this type of epilepsy.

Side effects can include:

Sedation, dizziness, and irritability
GI distress
Rash

Extreme caution should be used with:

Hepatic or renal disease
Pregnancy and lactation

See Table 22.1 for a summary of the anticonvulsants.

TABLE 22.1. ANTICONVULSANTS

Generic Name	Trade Name	Dosage	Comments
phenytoin	Dilantin	PO 300–600 mg qd in divided doses IM 100–200 mg q4h IV 150–250 mg	For grand mal, psychomotor, and focal epileptic seizures; frequently combined with phenobarbital; also used for digitalis-induced cardiac arrhythmias
primidone	Mysoline	PO 0.75–2 g qd in divided doses	Few toxic side effects
trimethadione	Tridione	300 mg PO tid	For petit mal seizures
ethosuximide	Zarontin	PO 250 mg–1.5 g qd in divided doses	For petit mal seizures

> **PATIENT EDUCATION**
>
> Patients taking any anticonvulsant medication should be instructed regarding:
>
> Caution with driving or operating machinery, until regulated with the medication, because of drowsiness or dizziness
>
> Reporting of any side effects, such as rash or eye problems, staggering, slurred speech, and any other symptoms
>
> Careful oral hygiene until tenderness of the gums subsides as treatment progresses
>
> Always taking medication on time and *never* omitting dosage (abrupt withdrawal of medication can lead to status epilepticus)
>
> Wearing Medic-Alert tag or bracelet at all times in case of accident or injury
>
> Taking medication with food or milk to lessen stomach upset

Antiparkinsonian Drugs

Antiparkinsonian drugs are usually given for Parkinson's disease, a chronic neurologic disorder characterized by muscle tremors, rigidity and weakness of muscles, and slowness of movement (bradykinesia). There is no cure for Parkinson's disease, and the treatment goal is to relieve symptoms and maintain mobility.

LEVODOPA

Levodopa (L-dopa) is the drug of choice for long-term treatment. Sinemet (a combination of levodopa and carbidopa) is most often used.

Side effects include:

Nausea, vomiting, and anorexia
Behavioral and neurological changes
Hypotension
Palpitations and cardiac arrhythmias

Contraindications include:

Bronchial asthma
COPD (chronic obstructive pulmonary disease)
Cardiac disease or hypotension
Active peptic ulcer
Diabetes
Glaucoma
Psychoses

Interactions may occur with:

Antihypertensives, which may potentiate hypotensive effect

Phenytoin, which antagonizes levodopa

Vitamin B_6 (pyridoxine), which antagonizes levodopa alone but does not effect action of Sinemet

MAO inhibitors, which may cause hypertensive crisis

Patients receiving levodopa for prolonged periods of time may develop a tolerance, resulting in ineffectiveness of the drug. To prevent or treat this late failure of levodopa, a semisynthetic drug, bromocriptine (Parlodel) has sometimes been added to the treatment regimen for parkinsonian syndrome. Addition of bromocriptine allows a gradual reduction in the dosage of levodopa. Bromocriptine is not generally used alone in treatment because of a high incidence of adverse side effects.

Side effects of bromocriptine can include:

Psychosis, hallucinations, and confusion

Hypotension

Nausea

ANTICHOLINERGIC AGENTS

Drugs with anticholinergic and antihistaminic actions were the first to be used for parkinsonism and are still useful in mild forms of the disease and for drug-induced parkinsonism. The anticholinergics include synthetic atropinelike drugs, such as Artane and Cogentin, which are used to prevent or treat parkinsonlike tremors associated with long-term use of the major tranquilizers or for other forms of parkinsonian syndrome.

Side effects of the atropinelike drugs (anticholinergic in action) are:

Dry mouth

Dizziness and drowsiness

Blurred vision

Constipation

Urinary retention

Hypotension

AMANTADINE

Another drug unrelated to the other antiparkinson agents is amantadine (Symmetrel). It is used to treat parkinsonism (extrapyramidal reactions) associated with prolonged use of phenothiazines, carbon monoxide poisoning, or cerebral arteriosclerosis in the elderly.

Side effects of Symmetrel, usually dose related and reversible, can include:

Psychic disturbances, including depression, confusion, hallucinations, anxiety, irritability, and nervousness
Headache, weakness, and insomnia
Congestive heart failure, edema, and hypotension
GI distress, constipation, and urinary retention

Contraindications or extreme caution applies to:

Liver and kidney disease
Cardiac disorders
Psychosis, neurosis, and mental depression
Epilepsy
Patients taking CNS drugs

PATIENT EDUCATION

Patients taking antiparkinson drugs should be instructed regarding:

Administration on a regular schedule as prescribed, with food to lessen GI distress
Avoiding abrupt withdrawal of medication, which may greatly increase parkinsonian symptoms
Several weeks sometimes being required before benefit is apparent
Caution with CNS drugs, alcohol, or antihypertensives (not taking other medicines without physician approval)
Caution with driving or operation of machinery; drugs may cause drowsiness, dizziness, or lightheadedness
Reporting adverse side effects to the physician (e.g., blurred vision, constipation, urinary retention, GI symptoms, palpitations, and mental changes)
Reporting any signs that the drug is no longer effective after prolonged use (sometimes after months or years, the dosage may need to be increased or another drug substituted by the physician); avoiding any changes without medical supervision
Maintaining physical activity, self-care, and social interaction, an essential part of therapy for Parkinson's disease

---

See Table 22.2 for a summary of the antiparkinson's drugs.

TABLE 22.2. ANTIPARKINSONIAN DRUGS

Generic Name	Trade Name	Dosage	Comments
levodopa	L-dopa	PO 3–8 gm qd	*Most effective* for nondrug-induced parkinsonism; delayed onset of action
levodopa and carbidopa	Sinemet	25–250 mg given in divided dosage	Terminiate levodopa at least 8 h before Sinemet
bromocriptine	Parlodel	1.25–2.5 mg bid	Used with levodopa, dosage gradually increased to optimum maintenance dose
anticholinergics			
benztropin	Cogentin	PO, IM, or IV 0.5–6 mg qd in one or divided doses	For drug-induced parkinsonism and other forms of parkinsonian syndrome
trihexyphenidyl	Artane	PO 1–15 mg qd in divided doses	For drug-induced parkinsonism and other forms of parkinsonian syndrome
amantadine	Symmetrel	100–300 mg qd DD	Also for viral upper respiratory infection and drug-induced parkinsonism

WORKSHEET FOR CHAPTER 22

Anticonvulsants and Antiparkinson's Drugs

List the drugs according to category and complete all columns.

CLASSIFICATIONS AND DRUGS	PURPOSE	SIDE EFFECTS	CONTRAINDICATIONS OR CAUTIONS	PATIENT EDUCATION
Anticonvulsants 1. 2. 3.				
Antiparkinsonian Drugs with Levodopa 1. L-dopa 2. Sinemet				
Anticholinergics for Parkinson's 1. 2.				
Amantadine 1. Symmetrel				

23

Endocrine System Drugs

OBJECTIVES

Upon completion of this chapter, the student will be able to:

1. Identify the hormones secreted by these four endocrine glands: pituitary, adrenals, thyroid, and islets of Langerhans.
2. Describe at least five conditions that can be treated with corticosteroids.
3. Explain administration practice important to corticosteroid therapy.
4. List at least four serious potential side effects of long-term steroid therapy.
5. Compare and contrast medications given for hypothyroidism and hyperthyroidism.
6. Describe side effects of thyroid and antithyroid agents.
7. Explain uses and side effects of oral hypoglycemics.
8. Compare and contrast insulins according to action (rapid, intermediate, and long acting), naming onset, peak, and duration of each category.
9. Identify the symptoms of hypoglycemia and hyperglycemia, and appropriate interventions.
10. Explain appropriate patient education for those receiving endocrine system drugs.

Endocrine system drugs include natural hormones secreted by the ductless glands or synthetic substitutes. Hormones that affect the reproductive system are discussed in Chapter 24. This chapter covers four categories: pituitary hormones, adrenal corticosteroids, thyroid agents, and antidiabetic agents.

Pituitary Hormones

The pituitary gland, located at the base of the brain, is called the master gland because it regulates the function of the other glands. It secretes four hormones: somatotropin, adrenocorticotropic hormone (ACTH), thyroid-stimulating hormone (TSH), and gonadotropic hormones (FSH, LH, and LTH; see Chapter 24). The two pituitary hormones discussed in this chapter are somatotropin and ACTH.

SOMATOTROPIN

Somatotropin (Asellacrin) is the drug obtained by extracting the human growth hormone, somatotropin, from human pituitary glands. It is used to promote linear growth in patients with growth failure. Intramuscular injections are given weekly or three times per week for 6 months to 1 year, with dosage regulated by response to therapy.

Side effects, which are rare and usually subside within 1–2 months, may include:

Pain at injection site
Hypercalciuria

Contraindications or extreme caution applies to:

Brain tumor
Patients not showing response within 1 year
Diabetic patients

PATIENT EDUCATION

Patients should be instructed regarding:

Importance of treatment under the supervision of a physician specializing in endocrine deficiency disorders
Necessity of prolonged treatment, from 6 months to 1 year
Reporting any urinary symptoms

Interactions include:

Potentiation with thyroid agents and androgens (may cause early closure of
bone ends, which stops growth)
Antagonism by corticosteroids

ACTH

Adrenocorticotropic hormone is available *only for parenteral use,* mainly in the
diagnosis of adrenocortical insufficiency. At times ACTH is also prescribed for its
anti-inflammtory properties as ACTHar gel (the vial must be warmed in water
to liquify the gel for injection). However, the corticosteroids are usually preferable for therapy because dosage can be regulated more accurately with them
and corticosteroids are available in oral form.

Side effects of ACTH on a *short-term* basis are rare but may include hypersensitivity reactions (e.g., rash, vertigo, fever, wheezing, and anaphylaxis). *Long-
term* use of ACTH is *not* recommended because of many serious side effects
comparable to the effects of corticosteroid therapy (see next section).

Adrenal Corticosteroids

The adrenal glands, located adjacent to the kidneys, secrete hormones called
corticosteroids, which act by *suppressing the body's response to infection or trauma.*
They *relieve inflammation, reduce swelling* and *suppress symptoms* in acute conditions. Corticosteroid use can be subdivided into two broad categories: (1) as
replacement therapy when secretions of the pituitary or adrenal glands are deficient and (2) for their antiinflammatory and immunosupspressive properties.
   Corticosteroid therapy is *not curative,* but is used as *supportive therapy with
other medications.* Some conditions treated on a *short-term* basis with corticosteroids include:

Allergic reactions (e.g., to insect bites, poison plants, chemicals or other medications), in which there are symptoms of rash, hives, or anaphylaxis.
Acute flare-ups of rheumatic or collagen disorders, especially where only a few
inflamed joints can be injected with corticosteroids to decrease crippling,
or in life-threatening situations, such as rheumatic carditis or lupus.
Acute flare-ups of severe skin conditions that do not respond to conservative therapy; topical applications are preferable to systemic therapy, when possible,
to minimize side effects.
Acute respiratory disorders, such as status asthmaticus, sarcoidosis, or hyaline
membrane disease.
Malignancies (e.g., leukemia, lymphoma, and Hodgkin's disease), in which
corticosteroids (e.g., prednisone) are used with other antineoplastic drugs
as part of the chemotherapy regimen.

Cerebral edema associated with brain tumor, neurosurgery, or trauma.

Organ transplant, in which corticosteroids are used with other immunosuppressive drugs to prevent rejection of transplanted organs.

Life-threatening shock, in which corticosteroids (e.g., Decadron) in massive doses are given IV for 24–48 h maximum.

Prolonged administration of corticosteroids can cause suppression of the pituitary gland with adrenocortical atrophy, and the body no longer produces its own hormone. To minimize this effect, corticosteroids are given by *alternate-day* therapy when they are required for extended time periods. Withdrawal of corticosteroids following long-term therapy should always be gradual with *step-down* (i.e., tapering) dosage. Abrupt withdrawal can lead to acute adrenal insufficiency and even death.

Because of potentially serious side effects, corticosteroids are administered for as short a time as possible and *locally if possible* to reduce systemic effects (e.g., in ointment, intra-articular injections, ophthalmic drops, and respiratory aerosol inhalants).

Side effects of the corticosteroids, used for longer than very brief periods, can be *quite serious* and possibly include:

Adrenocortical insufficiency

Delayed wound healing and *increased susceptibility to infection*

Fluid and electrolyte imbalance, possibly resulting in edema, potassium loss, hypertension, and congestive heart failure

Muscle pain or weakness

Osteoporosis

Stunting of growth in children (premature closure of bone ends)

Increased intraocular pressure or cataracts

Endocrine disorders, including cushingoid state, amenorrhea, and *hyperglycemia*

Nausea, vomiting, diarrhea, and constipation

Gastric or esophageal irritation or *ulceration*

CNS effects, including headache, vertigo, insomnia, and euphoria

Petechiae and easy bruising

Contraindications or extreme caution applies to:

Long-term use (regulated carefully)

Viral or bacterial infections (used only in life-threatening situations)

Fungal infections (only if specific therapy concurrent)

Hypothyroidism or cirrhosis (exaggerated response to corticosteroids)

Hypertension or congestive heart failure

Psychotic patients

Diabetes (drugs increase hyperglycemia)

Glaucoma (drugs may increase intraocular pressure)

History of gastric or esophageal irritation (may precipitate ulcers)

Children (drugs may retard growth)

Pregnancy and lactation

Interactions may occur with:

Barbiturates, phenytoin (Dilantin), and rifampin

Estrogen may potentiate corticosteroids

Nonsteroidal anti-inflammatory agents (e.g., aspirin may increase risk of GI ulceration or salicylate intoxication)

Thiazide diuretics, which potentiate potassium depletion

Vaccines and toxoids (corticosteroids inhibit antibody response)

PATIENT EDUCATION

Patients should be instructed regarding:

Following exact dosage and administration orders (never taking longer than indicated and *never stopping medicine abruptly*)

Notifying physician of any signs of infection or trauma *while taking corticosteroids or within 12 months after long-term therapy is discontinued* and similarly notifying surgeon, dentist, or anesthesiologist if required

Taking oral corticosteroids during or immediately after meals to decrease gastric irritation

Avoiding any other drugs at same time (including OTC drugs, e.g., aspirin) without physician's approval

Side effects to expect with long-term therapy (e.g., fluid retention and edema)

See Table 23.1 for a summary of the pituitary drugs and adrenal corticosteroids.

TABLE 23.1. PITUITARY DRUGS AND ADRENAL CORTICOSTEROIDS

Generic Name	Trade Name	Dosage
Pituitary Drugs		
adrenocorticotropic hormone (ACTH)	ACTHar	IM sol, gel, suspension 40 U q12–24h
somatropin	Asellacrin	IM 2–6 IU 3 ×/week
Adrenal Corticosteroids[a]		
dexamethasone	Decadron	PO, IV, IM, topical injections
hydrocortisone	Cortef or Solu-Cortef	PO, IV, IM
methylprednisolone	Medrol or Solu-Medrol	PO, IV, IM
prednisone	Prednisone	PO tabs or sol

[a]Dosage varies greatly, depending on the condition treated; massive doses are given for acute conditions on a short-term basis; long-term therapy is usually alternate-day, and dosage is reduced gradually.

Thyroid Agents

Thyroid agents can be natural (Thyroid) or synthetic (e.g., Synthroid). Thyroid preparations are used in replacement therapy for hypothyroidism caused by diminished or absent thyroid function. Hypothyroid conditions requiring replacement therapy include *cretinism* (congenital; requires immediate treatment to prevent mental retardation) and *myxedema* (adult hypothyroidism) due to lack of iodine in the diet, thyroid and pituitary disorders, and thyroid destruction from surgery or radiation. Hypothyroidism causes slowed metabolism with symptoms ranging from fatigue, dry skin, weight gain, sensitivity to cold, and irregular menses to mental deterioration if untreated.

Hypothyroidism is diagnosed by blood tests (e.g., T-3, T-4) or radioactive iodine uptake tests before medication is given. The use of thyroid agents in weight reduction programs to increase metabolism when thyroid function is normal (euthyroid), is *contraindicated* and dangerous, leading to decrease in normal thyroid function and possibly life-threatening cardiac arrhythmias.

Transient hypothyroidism is rare, and thyroid replacement therapy for true hypothyroidism must be continued for life, although dosage adjustments may be required.

Toxic effects are the result of overdosage of thyroid and are manifested in the signs of *hyperthyroidism:*

Palpitations, tachycardia, cardiac arrhythmias, and increased blood pressure
Nervousness, tremor, headache, and insomnia
Weight loss, diarrhea, and abdominal cramps
Intolerance to heat, fever, and excessive sweating
Menstrual irregularities

Contraindications or extreme caution applies to:

Cardiovascular disease, including angina pectoris and hypertension
Elderly persons (may precipitate dormant cardiac pathology)
Adrenal insufficiency
Diabetes
Euthyroid persons

PATIENT EDUCATION

Patients should be instructed regarding:

Importance of taking the prescribed dosage of medication consistently every day
Importance of reporting any symptoms of overdose (e.g., palpitations, nervousness, excessive sweating, and unexplained weight loss)
Periodic laboratory tests to determine effectiveness and proper dosage

---

Interactions of thyroid may occur with:

Potentiation of oral anticoagulant effects
Insulin and oral hypoglycemics (dosage adjustment necessary)
Potentiation of adrenergic effect (e.g., epinephrine)

Antithyroid Agents

Antithyroid agents (e.g., Tapazole and Propylthiouracil) are used *to relieve the symptoms of hyperthyroidism* in preparation for surgical or radioactive iodine therapy.

Side effects are rare and may include:

Rash, urticaria, and pruritis
Blood dyscracias (especially agranulocytosis)

Contraindications or caution applies to:

Prolonged therapy (seldom used)
Patients older than 40 years old
Pregnancy and lactation

Interactions with other drugs causing agranulocytosis are potentiated.

PATIENT EDUCATION

Patients should be instructed to notify the physician immediately of signs of illness (e.g., chills, fever, rash, sore throat, malaise, and jaundice).

See Table 23.2 for a summary of thyroid and antithyroid agents.

TABLE 23.2. THYROID AND ANTITHYROID AGENTS

Generic Name	Trade Name	Dosage
Thyroid Agents		
levothyroxin	Synthroid	100–400 mg qd
thyroid	Thyroid	60 mg qd
Antithyroid Agents		
methimazole	Tapazole	tabs, 5–15 mg qd
propylthiouracil	Propylthiouracil	tabs, 150 mg q8h

Antidiabetic Agents

Antidiabetic agents (hypoglycemics) are administered *to lower blood glucose levels* in those with impaired metabolism of carbohydrates, fats, and proteins. Diabetes are classified as type I (insulin dependent) or type II (non–insulin-dependent), formerly described as maturity-onset diabetes because type II is only found in adults over 40 years of age. However, adults sometimes develop type I diabetes.

INSULIN

Insulin is required as replacement therapy for type I diabetics with insufficient production of insulin from the islets of Langerhans in the pancreas. Insulin to treat type I diabetics must be administered parenterally because it is destroyed in the GI tract. In the past, insulins were prepared only from beef or pork pancreas. A newer form of insulin, called *insulin human* because its structure is identical to human insulin, is prepared in one of two ways in the laboratory:

1. *Biosynthetic* preparation includes a complex series of scientific steps in which cultures of *Escherichia coli* are modified by a process known as *recombinant DNA technology* to produce such insulins as Humulin R (regular) and Humulin N (isophane).
2. Semisynthetic preparation involves purifying or modifying pork insulin to produce such insulins as Actrapid (regular) and Monotard (zinc).

Biosynthetic insulin human (Humulin) is preferred to insulins from animal sources in patients with systemic allergic reactions, in some patients who are very difficult to regulate, or during pregnancy. Insulin human tends to peak sooner than the animal insulins, and therefore smaller amounts are required by some patients.

Most of the insulin used today is U-100, which means that there are 100 U of insulin in each milliliter. The insulin syringe *must be marked U-100* to match the insulin used.

Insulin preparations differ mainly in their onset, peak, and duration of action (Table 23.3). *Regular* insulin is rapid-acting and of short duration. Regular insulin is the only type that may be given intravenously as well as subcutaneously. The other insulins, which can only be given subcutaneously, include *isophane* (NPH) or Lente, which are intermediate acting; and *protamine zinc* (PZI) and Ultralente, which are long acting.

Regular insulin is sometimes combined with isophane or zinc insulin in the same syringe. When two insulins are ordered at the same time, the *regular* insulin should be drawn into the syringe first.

Regular insulin is sometimes ordered on a sliding scale. This means that the urine or blood is tested for sugar and a specific amount of regular insulin is administered SC based on the level of sugar shown by the test. For example, the physician may issue a standing order for insulin as needed according to glucosuria or high blood glucose.

When a urine test is used, the urine tested should be a fresh, double-voided specimen. The order might specify to give regular insulin, U-100, according to the following scale:

4+ urine glucose	20 U SC
3+ urine glucose	15 U SC
2+ urine glucose	10 U SC
1+ urine glucose	5 U SC

When a blood test is used, check blood glucose with fingerstick. The order might specify to give regular insulin, U-100, according to the following scale:

400 mg	15 U SC
300–400 mg	12 U SC
250–300 mg	8 U SC
180–250 mg	5 U SC

The actual insulin dose prescribed by the physician will vary with the individual patient. This is just an example of a possible prescription. Be sure to check the medication order carefully before administering any insulin.

TABLE 23.3. INSULINS

Beef or Pork	Synthetics	Action	Onset (h)	Peak Hours	Duration (h)
Regular	Humulin R,[a] Actrapid[b]	Rapid acting	½–1	2–3	5–7
Isophane (NPH) Lente	Humulin N[a]	Intermediate acting	1–2	8–12	18–24
Protamine zinc (PZI) Ultralente	Monotard[b]	Long acting	4–8	14–20	36

Note: This is a representative list. Other insulin products are also available. Dosage varies. Before giving insulin, always check expiration date on the vial, and be sure that regular insulins are clear and isophane and zinc insulins are cloudy. *Only regular* insulins may be administered IV. Isophane and zinc insulins are administered only SC, *never IV.*
[a]Biosynthetic insulin human.
[b]Semisynthetic insulin human.

Hyperglycemia or elevated blood glucose, may result from:

Undiagnosed diabetes
Insulin dose insufficiency
Infections
Surgical or other trauma
Emotional stress
Other endocrine disorders
Pregnancy

Symptoms of hyperglycemia may include:

Dehydration and excessive thirst
Anorexia and unexplained weight loss in persons under 40 years old
Polyuria (frequent urination)
Air hunger (Kussmaul's respiration) sighing respiration
Fruity breath
Lethargy, weakness, flu symptoms, and coma if untreated
Vision problems

Treatment of acute hyperglycemia (ketoacidosis) includes:

IV fluids to correct electrolyte imbalance
Regular insulin added to IV fluids

Interactions of insulin with *potentiation* of hypoglycemic effect include:

Alcohol
MAO inhibitors
Salicylates

Hypoglycemia, or lowered blood glucose (insulin reaction), may result from:

Overdose of insulin
Delayed or insufficient food intake (e.g., dieting)
Excessive or unusual exercise

Symptoms of hypoglycemia include:

Increased perspiration
Irritability and confusion
Tremor, weakness, and headache
Blurred or double vision
Loss of consciousness and convulsions if untreated

Treatment of hypoglycemia includes:

If conscious, administration of 4 oz orange juice, candy, honey, or syrup (especially sublingual)
If comatose, administration of 10–50 ml of 50% dextrose solution IV or administration of 0.5–1 U of glucagon (1 mg) IM or IV

ORAL HYPOGLYCEMICS

Patients with type II, non–insulin-dependent diabetes may sometimes be treated with diet alone or a combination of a low-calorie, low-fat, low-carbohydrate diet and oral hypoglycemics (e.g., Diabinese, Tolinase, and Orinase), structurally known as sulfonylureas.

Symptoms of type II diabetes may include:

Excessive weight gain after age 40
Excessive thirst (polydipsia)
Excessive urination (polyuria)
Excessive weakness, poor circulation, and slow healing
Visual problems

Side effects of oral hypoglycemics may include:

GI distress (may subside with dosage regulation)
Dermatologic effects, including pruritis, rash, and urticaria
Hepatic dysfunction, including jaundice (rare)
Weakness, fatigue, lethargy, vertigo, and headache
Blood dyscracias, including anemia
Hypoglycemia
Increased risk of cardiovascular death reported but not fully confirmed

Contraindications or extreme caution applies to:

Debilitated or malnourished patients
Impaired liver and kidney function
Unstable diabetes or type I diabetes
Major surgery, severe infection, and severe trauma

Interactions may include:

Alcohol, with a facial flushing, especially with Diabinese
Salicylates and other nonsteroidal anti-inflammatory agents
Oral anticoagulants, which are antagonistic
Thiazide diuretics, which may require increase in dose of hypoglycemic

See Table 23.4 for a summary of the oral hypoglycemics.

TABLE 23.4. ORAL HYPOGLYCEMICS

Generic Name	Trade Name	Dosage
chlorpropamide	Diabinese	100–250 mg qd
tolazamide	Tolinase	100–150 mg qd
tolbutamide	Orinase	250 mg–2 g qd

PATIENT EDUCATION

Both types of diabetics should be instructed regarding:

Early detection and treatment of hypoglycemia

Properly balanced diet (i.e., restricted calories; avoidance of sugar, sweets, and alcohol; reduced fats, high bulk; and sufficient fluids)

Regular exercise

Importance of reporting to a physician *immediately* if nausea, vomiting, diarrhea, or infections occur (IV fluids may be required to prevent dehydration and acidosis)

Good foot care to reduce chance of infections

Carrying identification card and wearing identification tag

For type I diabetics (those requiring insulin), the foregoing instructions are important, as well as these additional rules:

Rotate injection sites (Fig. 23.1).

Maintain aseptic technique with injections.

Keep insulin from excessive heat or freezing (keep at room temperature; use a wide-mouth Thermos when traveling)

Insulin dosage may sometimes be adjusted slightly, *if the physician agrees*, by following these rules:

- Increase insulin with illness, stress, or trauma.
- Reduce insulin with more exercise or less food.
- Check urine or blood glucose as directed by the physician.
- Have someone check the amount of insulin in the syringe before injection, especially with the elderly or those with vision impairment (retinal problems are common in diabetics).
- Check all insulin for expiration date.
- Check regular insulin for clearness; do *not* give if cloudy or discolored.
- Rotate isophane and zinc insulin vials to mix contents; do *not* give if solution is clear or clumped in appearance after rotation; do *not* shake the vial; rotate gently between hands (Fig. 23.2).

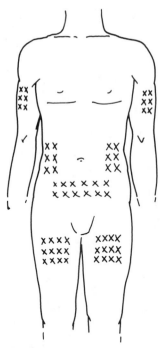

Figure 23.1 Common sites for insulin injection. Sites should be rotated.

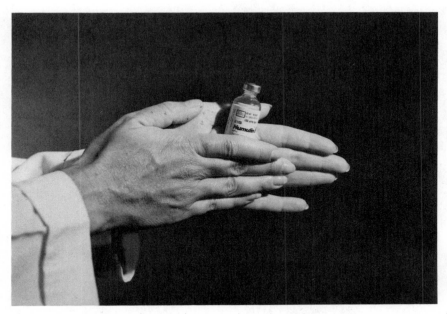

Figure 23.2 Rotate isophane and zinc insulin vials gently to mix contents. Do not shake.

WORKSHEET 1 FOR CHAPTER 23

Endocrine System Drugs

List the drugs according to category and complete all columns. Learn generic or trade names as specified by instructor.

CLASSIFICATIONS AND DRUGS	PURPOSE	SIDE EFFECTS	CONTRAINDICATIONS OR CAUTIONS	PATIENT EDUCATION
Corticosteroids				
1. Decadron				
2. Solu-Medrol				
3. prednisone				
Thyroid Agents				
1. Synthroid				
2. Thyroid				
Antithyroid Agents				
1. Tapazole				
2. Propylthiouracil				
Oral Hypoglycemics				
1. Diabinese				
2. Tolinase				
3. Orinase				

Note: Pituitary agents are given infrequently and are thus not included.

WORKSHEET 2 FOR CHAPTER 23

Insulins

Fill in the blanks and complete all columns. Learn generic or trade names as specified by instructor.

Regular, Humulin R: rapid acting, peak _____ h

NPH, Lente, Humulin N: intermediate acting, peak _____ h

PZI, Ultralente: long acting, peak _____ h

HYPERGLYCEMIA	CAUSES	SYMPTOMS	TREATMENT

HYPOGLYCEMIA	CAUSES	SYMPTOMS	TREATMENT

24

Reproductive System Drugs

OBJECTIVES

Upon completion of this chapter, the student will be able to:

1. Identify the uses, side effects, and precautions for the androgens.
2. List the uses, side effects, and contraindications for the estrogens and progesterone.
3. Describe the use of oxytocics and the precautions to be observed.
4. Explain the use of ritodrine and terbutaline.
5. Describe contraceptive products and use.
6. Given a list of drugs associated with the reproductive system, categorize according to use.
7. Explain appropriate patient education for representative drugs in each category.

Hormones that regulate the functions of the reproductive systems include *endogenous* chemical substances, which originate within different areas of the body. For the purpose of simplification, we will divide the reproductive hormones into four main categories: gonadotropic, androgens, estrogens, and progestins.

The pituitary gland is located at the base of the brain. The anterior lobe secretes four hormones. Those affecting growth, thyroid function, and adrenocorticosteroid production are discussed in Chapter 23. This chapter includes the gonadotropic hormones, which are secreted by the anterior and posterior pituitary lobes.

The gonadotropic hormones include (1) follicle-stimulating hormone (FSH), which stimulates development of ovarian follicles in the female and sperm production in the testes of the male; (2) luteinizing hormone (LH), which works in conjunction with FSH to induce secretion of estrogen, ovulation, and development of corpus luteum; and (3) luteotropic hormone (LTH), which stimulates the secretion of progesterone by the corpus luteum and secretion of milk by the mammary gland, hence the term lactogenic hormone.

Androgens

Androgens, the male hormones, are secreted mainly in the interstitial tissue of the testes in the male and secondarily in the adrenal glands of both sexes. Androgens, which stimulate the development of male characteristics (masculinization), include testosterone and andosterone. Inadequate production of androgens in the male may be due to pituitary malfunction; or atrophy, injury to, or removal of the testicles (castration), resulting in eunuchoidism. Eunuchoid characteristics include retarded development of sex organs, absence of beard and bodily hair, high-pitched voice, and lack of muscular development. Hypogonadism may also result in impotence or deficient sperm production (oligospermia).

Uses of androgens, such as methyltestosterone (oral) and testosterone (parenteral), include:

1. *Replacement* in cases of diminished testicular hormone (e.g., with impotence or oligospermia)
   Congenital hypogonadism (e.g., cryptorchidism or undescended testicles) or delayed puberty in the male
   Acquired hypogonadism (e.g., orchitis, trauma, tumor, radiation, or surgery of the testicles)
2. *Palliative treatment* of females with advanced metastatic (skeletal) carcinoma of the breast
   Endometriosis and fibrocystic breast disease
   Prevention of postpartum breast engorgement in *nonnursing* mothers (usually combined with estrogen)

Side effects can include:

Edema (diuretics may be indicated)
Acne

TABLE 24.1. ANDROGENS

Generic Name	Trade Name	Dosage	Comments
danazol	Danocrine	PO 100–800 mg qd	For endometriosis, fibrocystic breast disease
methyltestosterone	Android, Testred	PO 10–50 mg qd, buccal 5–25 mg qd	For male hypogonadism
		PO 50–200 mg qd, buccal 25–100 mg qd	For advanced breast cancer
testosterone	Depo-Testosterone	Deep IM, dosage varies; pellet implant, SC	For hypogonadism, advanced breast cancer
testosterone in combination with estrogen	Deladumone	IM 25–50 mg qd × 3–4	For breast engorgement

Oligospermia (deficient sperm production)

Increased or decreased sexual stimulation or libido

Gynecomastia in males (enlarged breast tissue)

Hirsutism, deepening of voice, and amenorrhea in females

Jaundice and hepatitis

Nausea and vomiting

Premature closure of bone ends in adolescents, with stunting of growth

Contraindications or caution applies to:

Cardiac, renal, and liver dysfunction (edema common)

Geriatric males (may increase risk of prostatic hypertrophy and carcinoma or overstimulation sexually)

Prepubertal males who have not reached their full growth potential (may stunt growth)

Interactions may occur with:

Oral anticoagulants (potentiation may cause bleeding)

Decreased blood glucose and decreased insulin requirements in diabetics

---

PATIENT EDUCATION

Patients should be instructed regarding:

Side effects to report, especially edema, jaundice, nausea, or vomiting

Sexual effects for males to report, such as decreased ejaculatory volume and excessive sexual stimulation, especially in geriatric patients beyond cardiovascular capacity

Sexual effects for females to expect (e.g., hirsutism and voice deepening)

Possibility of stunted growth when administered to adolescent boys before puberty

---

See Table 24.1 for a summary of the androgens.

Estrogens

Estrogens, the female sex hormones, are produced mainly by the ovary and secondarily by the adrenal glands. Estrogens are responsible for the development of female secondary sexual characteristics, including breast enlargement, and during the menstrual cycle act on the female genitalia to produce an environment suitable for fertilization, implantation, and nutrition of the early embryo. Estrogens also affect the secretion of the hormones FSH and LH from the anterior pituitary gland in a complex way. This results in inhibition of lactation and inhibition of ovulation, the latter process utilized in contraceptive therapy.

Uses of estrogen therapy include:

Contraception (usually combined wtih progestin)
Menopausal vasomotor symptom relief (*not* effective against depression or nervous symptoms)
Female hypogonadism due to ovarian pathology or oophorectomy
Postmenopausal prevention of osteoporosis (calcium depletion) and atrophic vaginitis from decreased secretions
Inhibition of lactation in nonnursing mothers
Postcoital use after rape or incest (within 24–48 h) of a single large dose to prevent, not terminate, pregnancy

Side effects of estrogen therapy, especially with high doses, can include:

Possible thromboembolic disorderes and increased risk of myocardial infarction
GI effects, including vomiting, abdominal cramps, bloating, diarrhea, and weight gain
Skin discolorations (acne may decrease or occasionally increase)
Elevated blood pressure
Fluid retention and edema
Increased serum triglyceride levels
Severe hypercalcemia in cancer patients with large doses
Folic acid deficiency (may require folic acid supplements)
Liver function abnormalities, including jaundice, anorexia, and pruritis
Breakthrough or irregular vaginal bleeding
Increased risk of cervical erosion and *Candida* vaginitis
Headache, especially migraine
Visual disturbances
Breast tenderness, enlargement, and secretion
Increased risk of gallbladder disease

Contraindications and precautions exist because the use of estrogens, especially in large doses, may be associated with increased risk of several serious conditions. Before estrogen therapy is begun, a complete history and physical examination are essential, and yearly physicals during therapy are important. Estrogens are *contraindicated* for anyone with a history of the following conditions, and estrogen therapy should be *discontinued with signs of these conditions:*

Thromboembolus, stroke, and myocardial infarction
Liver dysfunction and gallbladder disease
Visual disturbances, severe headaches, and migraine
Hypertension, shortness of breath, and chest or calf pain
Seizure, asthma, and kidney disorders
Surgery (estrogens should be discontinued 4 weeks before if possible)
Breast nodules, fibrocystic disease, abnormal mammography, or family history of breast cancer

Other contraindications include the following:

Prolonged continued use of estrogens in postmenopausal women, which has shown an increased risk of endometrial cancer in some studies; therefore, cyclic administration at the *lowest* possible dose is recommended with regular physical examinations, including a Pap test every year.
Pregnancy, in which estrogens can cause serious fetal toxicity, congenital anomalies, and vaginal or cervical cancer in later life. Estrogens should *never* be used to treat threatened abortions or if there is any possibility of pregnancy.
Nursing mothers should avoid estrogen.

Interactions include the following:

Rifampin and isoniazid decrease estrogenic activity, and therefore other forms of contraception should be used with patients receiving rifampin or isoniazid.
Corticosteroid effects are potentiated by estrogen.
Oral anticoagulant action is decreased by estrogen.
Laboratory test interference includes endocrine function tests, decreased glucose tolerance, and thyroid function tests
Anti-infectives may decrease contraceptive action.
Anticonvulsants, hypotensives, and oral hypoglycemic actions may be decreased or increased.

Progestins

Progesterone is a hormone secreted by the corpus luteum and adrenal glands. It is responsible for changes in uterine endometrium in the second half of the menstrual cycle in preparation for implantation of the fertilized ovum, development of maternal placenta after implantation, and development of mammary glands. Synthetic drugs that exert progesterone-like activity are called progestins.

Uses of synthetic progestins include:

Treatment of amenorrhea and abnormal uterine bleeding caused by hormonal imbalance

Contraception, usually combined with estrogen (not as effective as a contraceptive when used alone)

Adjunctive and palliative therapy for advanced and metastatic endometrial or renal cancer

Side effects of continuous progestin use can include:

Menstrual irregularity and amenorrhea
Breakthrough bleeding and spotting
Edema and weight gain
Nausea
Breast tenderness, enlargement, and secretion
Jaundice, rash, and pruritis
Headache and migraine
Mental depression
Cervical erosion
Thromboembolic disorders
Vision disorders

Contraindications and cautions with progestin (similar to cautions with estrogen) apply to:

Any condition that might be aggravated by fluid retention (e.g., asthma, seizures, migraine, and cardiac or renal dysfunction)

History of mental depression
History of thromboembolic disorders
History of cerebrovascular accident
Liver disorders
Undiagnosed vaginal bleeding
Pregnancy (progestins are no longer used to treat threatened abortion because of the potential adverse effects to the fetus)
Nursing mothers

See Table 24.2 for a summary of the estrogens and progestins.

TABLE 24.2. ESTROGENS AND PROGESTINS

Generic Name	Trade Name	Dosage	Comments
Estrogens			
chlorotrianisene	TACE	PO; dose varies with condition	For female hypogonadism, breast engorgement, prostate cancer
diethylstilbestrol	DES	PO, intravaginal; dose varies with condition	For female hypogonadism, breast engorgement, prostate cancer
conjugated estrogens	Premarin, others	PO, vaginal cream, parenteral; dose varies with condition	For female hypogonadism, breast engorgement, prostate cancer, menopausal symptoms
Progestins			
progesterone	Delalutin, Provera	Parenteral, PO, IM; dose varies with condition	For abnormal uterine bleeding, menopausal symptoms

Note: Estrogen-progestin oral contraceptive combinations are too numerous to mention. To ensure maximum contraceptive efficiency, medication must be taken *exactly* as prescribed and as near as possible to the same time each day.

PATIENT EDUCATION

Patients taking estrogen, progesterone, or combinations of the two should be instructed regarding:

Importance of following prescribed schedule with contraceptives

Taking with or after evening meal or at hs, same time every day

Minor adverse effects of contraceptives, which usually diminish or disappear after three to four cycles

Possible serious side effects and the importance of reporting any signs of cardiovascular or kidney disorders, liver or gallbladder dysfunction, rash, jaundice, GI symptoms, visual disturbance, severe headache, breast lumps, irregular vaginal bleeding, shortness of breath, and chest or calf pain

Regular breast self-examination

Complete physical examination including Pap test at least yearly

Avoidance of all estrogen or progestin products if pregnant or nursing

---

Drugs for Labor and Delivery

In addition to the hormones secreted by the anterior pituitary gland, there is also a hormone secreted by the posterior pituitary lobe: oxytocin. This hormone stimulates the uterus to contract, thus inducing childbirth. Oxytocin also acts on the mammary gland to stimulate the release of milk. Synthetic chemicals used to stimulate uterine contractions are called *oxytocics* and include oxytocin, prostaglandin, and ergonovine (Methergine or Ergotrate).

OXYTOCIN

Uses of oxytocin (IV infusion of dilute solutions slowly and at a carefully monitored rate) include:

Induction of labor with at-term or near-term pregnancies associated with hypertension (e.g., preeclampsia, eclampsia, or cardiovascular-renal disease), maternal diabetes, or uterine fetal death at term

Stimulating uterine contractions during the first or second stages of labor if labor is prolonged or if dysfunctional uterine inertia occurs

Pelvic adequacy and other maternal and fetal conditions must be evaluated carefully prior to induction of labor. Caesarian section may be preferable and safer in some instances

Side effects can be serious, resulting even in maternal or fetal death. *Extreme caution* with administration and *constant maternal* and *fetal monitoring* are required to prevent dangerous side effects such as:

Tetanic contractions with risk of uterine rupture

Cervical lacerations

Abruptio placenta

Impaired uterine blood flow

Amniotic fluid embolism

Fetal trauma, including intracranial hemorrhage

Fetal cardiac arrhythmias, including bradycardia, tachycardia, and premature ventricular contractions

Fetal death due to asphyxia

With large amounts of oxytocin, watch for:

Severe hypotension

Tachycardia and arrhythmias

Postpartum bleeding

Subarachnoid hemorrhage

Hypertensive episodes

Contraindications include:

Elective induction of labor merely for physician or patient convenience, which is *not* a valid indication for oxytocin use

Cephalopelvic disproportion, unfavorable fetal position, or presentation

Uterine or cervical scarring from major cervical or uterine surgery

Fetal distress when delivery is not imminent

Placenta previa, prolapsed cord, and multiparity

Prolonged use with severe toxemia

PROSTAGLANDIN

Uses (via intra-amniotic instillation) include:

Therapeutic abortion late in the second trimester (beyond the sixteenth week)

Uterine evacuation in cases of intrauterine fetal death in late pregnancy, benign hydatidiform mole, or fetuses with ancephaly, erythroblastosis fetalis, or other congenital abnormalities incompatible with life

Side effects can be minimized by administration of a prior test dose and symptomatic treatment of such effects as:

GI hypermotility, including nausea, vomiting, diarrhea, and abdominal cramping

Bradycardia, hypotension, hypertension, and arrhythmias

Dizziness, syncope, and flushing

Bronchospasm, including wheezing, dyspnea, chest constriction, and chest pain

Cervical laceration or uterine rupture (less common)

Retained placenta (less common)

Contraindications and precautions include:

Use only by physicians trained in amniocentesis and in a hospital where intensive care and surgical facilities are available

Contraindicated with history of pelvic surgery, uterine fibroids, and cervical stenosis

Caution with asthma, hypertension, cardiovascular disease, and epilepsy

ERGONOVINE

Uses of ergonovine (Ergotrate, Methergine) include prevention and treatment of postpartum and postabortion hemorrhage.

Side effects occur most commonly when administered IV undiluted or too rapidly or in conjunction with regional anesthesia or vasoconstrictors and can include:

Nausea and vomiting

Dizziness, headache, diaphoresis, palpitation, dyspnea, and arrhythmias

Hypertension (less common with Methergine)

Numbness and coldness of extremities with overdose

Contraindications and cautions include:

When administered during third stage of labor, may lead to retained placenta

Contraindicated with cardiovascular disease, especially hypertension, and with hepatic and renal impairment

RITODRINE AND TERBUTALINE

Drugs used to inhibit uterine contractions in premature labor include ritodrine and terbutaline. Prolongation of gestation may reduce the incidence of neonatal death and respiratory distress syndrome. These drugs are used only after a gestation period of 20–36 weeks, with regular contractions every 7–10 min, with amniotic membranes intact, and with cervical dilatation not more than 4 cm.

Side effects of ritodrine and terbutaline (adrenergics) are usually dose related and can include:

Increase in maternal and fetal heart rates with palpitations
Elevated blood glucose with glycosuria and keotacidosis
Tremor, nausea, vomiting, headache, irritability, anxiety, and chest pain

Contraindications or extreme caution applies to:

Cardiac disease and hypertension
Diabetes
Hyperthyroidism

MAGNESIUM SULFATE

Treatment of severe preeclampsia or eclampsia consists of magnesium sulfate ($MgSO_4$) injection for prevention and control of seizures. Magnesium sulfate acts by depressing the CNS and blocking neuromuscular transmission, thus producing anticonvulsant effects. Magnesium sulfate has also been used in the management of uterine tetany associated with the use of oxytocic agents. Magnesium sulfate also acts peripherally, producing vasodilation and lowering the blood pressure. Patients receiving this drug must be monitored closely for vital signs and reflexes.

Side effects, which can be serious and even fatal, can include:

Flaccid paralysis and CNS depression
Circulatory collapse, cardiac depression, and hypotension
Fatal respiratory paralysis
Flushing and sweating

The antidote for overdose of magnesium sulfate (e.g., respiratory depression or heart block) is IV administration of calcium gluconate.

Contraindications or extreme caution applies to:

Impaired renal function
Heart block or myocardial damage
Use more than 24 h before delivery and within 2 h of delivery because of potential respiratory depression in the neonate

See Table 24.3 for a summary of drugs for labor and delivery.

TABLE 24.3. DRUGS FOR LABOR AND DELIVERY

Generic Name	Trade Name	Dosage	Comments
Oxytocics[a]			
ergonovine	Ergotrate	PO, IM, IV; dosage varies	For postpartum hemorrhage
methylergonovine	Methergine	PO, IM, IV; dosage varies	For postpartum hemorrhage
oxytocin	Pitocin, Syntocinon	IV, nasal spray	For induction of labor, postpartum hemorrhage, promotion of milk ejection
Adrenergics[b]			
ritodrine HCl	Yutopar	IV, PO; dosage varies	
terbutaline sulfate	Brethine	IV, PO; dosage varies	
Treatment for Preeclampsia or Eclampsia			
magnesium sulfate	MgSO₄	IV; dosage varies	Watch for respiratory complications

[a]Stimulate uterine contractions.
[b]Inhibit uterine contractions in preterm labor.

WORKSHEET FOR CHAPTER 24

Reproductive System Drugs

List the drugs according to category and complete all columns. Learn generic or trade names as specified by instructor.

CLASSIFICATIONS AND DRUGS	PURPOSE	SIDE EFFECTS	CONTRAINDICATIONS OR CAUTIONS	PATIENT EDUCATION
Androgen				
1. testosterone				
Estrogens				
1. TACE				
2. diethylstilbestrol (DES)				
3. Premarin				
1. progesterone				
Oxytocics				
1. Ergotrate				
2. Methergine				
1. Magnesium sulfate				

25

Cardiovascular Drugs

OBJECTIVES

Upon completion of this chapter, the student will be able to:

1. Define cardiotonic, digitalization, cardioversion, bradycardia, tachycardia, hypotensive, ischemia, and hypoxia.
2. Describe the action and effects of digitalis and toxic side effects that require reporting.
3. Identify the different types of antiarrhythmics and the side effects of each.
4. Identify the most commonly used antihypertensives and the usual side effects, as well as the exceptions to the rule.
5. Describe the different types of coronary and peripheral vasodilators with cautions and side effects.
6. Name the two most commonly used vasoconstrictors and their purpose.
7. Compare and contrast heparin and coumarin derivatives in terms of administration, action, and antidotes.
8. Explain appropriate and important patient education for each of the six categories of cardiovascular drugs.

Cardiovascular drugs include medications that affect the heart and blood vessels as well as the anticoagulants. The drugs in this chapter are divided into six categories: cardiac glycosides, antiarrhythmic agents, antihypertensives, vasodilators, vasoconstrictors, and anticoagulants. Some of the drugs described in this chapter fall into more than one category because of multiple actions and uses (e.g., propranolol, which is used to treat cardiac arrhythmias, hypertension, and angina). Diuretics, which also affect the blood vessels and reduce blood pressure, are discussed in Chapter 15.

Cardiac Glycosides

Cardiac glycosides occur widely in nature or can be prepared synthetically. Cardiac glycosides have been called *cardiotonic* because they strengthen the heartbeat. These glycosides act directly on the myocardium to increase the force of myocardial contractions.

In patients with congestive heart failure, the heart fails to pump adequately to remove excess fluids from the pulmonary circulation, and pulmonary congestion results. The heart increases in size to compensate for the increased work load. Symptoms of congestive heart failure are dyspnea, cyanosis, increased heart rate, cough, and pitting edema.

In patients with congestive heart failure, the cardiac glycosides act by *increasing the force of the cardiac contractions*, thereby *increasing cardiac output.* As a result of increased efficiency, the *heart beats slower,* the heart size shrinks, and the diuretic action decreases edema.

The most commonly used cardiac glycosides are digitalis products. Of these, *digoxin* (Lanoxin) is used the most frequently because it can be administered orally and parenterally and has intermediate duration of action. *Digitoxin* (Crystodigin) has a prolonged action and the effects may persist for weeks.

Digitalization is the process of establishing the correct therapeutic dose of digitalis for maintaining optimal functioning of the heart without toxic effects. There is a very narrow margin between effective therapy and dangerous toxicity. Careful monitoring of cardiac function, side effects, and blood digitalis level is required to determine the therapeutic maintenance dose. Checking the apical pulse before administering digitalis is an important part of this monitoring process. If the apical pulse rate is less than 60, digitalis should be withheld until the physician is consulted. The action taken should be documented.

In emergency situations, deslanoside (Cedilanid-D) is administered intravenously for its rapid digitalizing effect. Modification of dosage is based on individual requirements and response, as determined by general condition, renal function, and cardiac function, monitored by electrocardiogram (ECG).

Toxic side effects of digitalis, which should be reported to the physician immediately, can include:

Anorexia, nausea, and vomiting (early signs of toxicity)
Abdominal cramping, distention, and diarrhea

Headache, fatigue, lethargy, and muscle weakness
Vertigo, restlessness, irritability, tremors, and seizures
Visual disturbances
Cardiac arrhythmias of all kinds, especially bradycardia (rate less than 60)
Gynecomastia with prolonged use in elderly men and women

Treatment of digitalis toxicity includes:

Discontinuing the drug immediately (usually sufficient)
Potassium chloride for arrhythmias if hypokalemia exists
Drugs such as atropine for severe bradycardia
Antiarrhythmics if indicated, especially phenytoin IV

Contraindications or extreme caution applies to:

Severe pulmonary disease
Hypothyroidism
Acute myocardial infarction
Acute myocarditis
Acute glomerulonephritis
Arrhythmias not caused by heart failure
Pregnancy and lactation

Interactions of digitalis may occur with:

Antacids, sulfa, neomycin, and anticholinergics reduce absorption of digitalis
  (administer far apart).
Diuretics and calcium can increase chance of arrhythmias.
Quinidine potentiates digitalis toxicity.
Adrenergics (epinephrine, ephedrine, and isoproterenol) increase the risk of
  arrhythmias.
Phenobarbital or phenytoin reduce digitalis levels.

PATIENT EDUCATION

Patients taking digitalis should be instructed regarding:

Recognition and immediate reporting of side effects
Holding medication, if any side effects occur, until the physician can be consulted
Avoiding taking any other medication at the same time
Avoiding all OTC medication, especially antacids and cold remedies

---

Antiarrhythmic Agents

Antiarrhythmic agents include a variety of drugs that act in different ways to suppress various types of cardiac arrhythmias, including atrial or ventricular tachycardias, atrial fibrillation or flutter, and arrhythmias that occur with digitalis toxicity or during surgery and anesthesia. The choice of a particular antiarrhythmic agent is based on careful assessment of many factors, including the type of arrhythmia; frequency; cardiac, renal, or other pathologic condition; and current signs and symptoms.

The role of the health care worker is vital in this area in accurate and timely reporting of vital signs and pertinent observations regarding effectiveness of medications and adverse side effects. Adequate knowledge of drug action and effects, and good judgment are essential.

Side effects of the individual medications are discussed separately. However, keep in mind that most of the drugs given to counteract arrhythmias have the potential for lowering blood pressure and slowing heartbeat. Therefore, it is especially important to be alert for signs of *hypotension* and *bradycardia*, which could lead to cardiac arrest. Although the antiarrhythmics commonly slow the heart rate, there are exceptions (e.g., procainamide and quinidine, which may cause *tachycardia*). When cardiac drugs are administered concomitantly, cardiac effects may be additive or antagonistic.

ADRENERGIC BLOCKERS

Adrenergic blockers, bretylium (Bretylol) and propranolol (Inderal), combat arrhythmias by inhibiting adrenergic (sympathetic) nerve receptors. The action is complex, and the results can include a vasodilating effect.

Bretylol is used most commonly in conjunction with cardioversion (electrical defibrillation) in patients unresponsive to other drugs. It has a delayed onset of antiarrhythmic action and frequently causes hypotension, and is therefore used only with constant ECG and blood pressure monitoring.

Propranolol (Inderal) is effective in the management of various cardiac arrhythmias. It is also used in the treatment of hypertension and some forms of chronic angina.

Side effects of propranolol, especially in patients over 60 years old and more commonly with IV administration of the drug, can include:

Hypotension, with vertigo and syncope

Bradycardia, with heart block and cardiac arrest

CNS symptoms (usually with long-term treatment with high doses), including dizziness, irritability, confusion, nightmares, insomnia, visual disturbances, and weakness

GI symptoms, including nausea, vomiting, and diarrhea

Rash or hematologic effects (rare or transient)

Bronchospasm, especially with history of asthma

Hypoglycemia

Contraindications or extreme caution applies to:

Withdrawal after prolonged use (should always be gradual)
Major surgery (withdrawal 48 h before surgery usually recommended)
Diabetes (causes hypoglycemia)
Renal and hepatic impairment
Asthma and allergic rhinitis
Bradycardia, heart block, and congestive heart failure
Pediatric use, pregnancy, and lactation

Interactions include antagonism of propranolol by:

Adrenergics (e.g., epinephrine and isoproterenol)
Anticholinergics
Tricyclic antidepressants

Potentiation of the effects of propranolol occur with:

Diuretics and other antihypertensives
Phenothiazine and other tranquilizers
Cimetidine (Tagamet), which slows metabolism of drug
Other cardiac drugs, which may potentiate toxic effects
Alcohol, muscle relaxants, and sedatives, which may precipitate hypotension, dizziness, confusion, or sedation

CALCIUM BLOCKERS

Calcium blockers, such as verapamil (Isoptin), counteract arrhythmias by suppressing the action of calcium in contraction of the heart muscle, thereby reducing cardiac excitability and dilating the main coronary arteries. Calcium blockers are also used in the treatment of angina and hypertension.

Side effects of verapamil can include:

Hypotension, with vertigo, headache
Bradycardia, with heart block
Constipation, nausea, and abdominal discomfort

Contraindications or extreme caution applies to:

Heart block and heart failure
Hepatic and renal impairment
Pregnancy and lactation

Interactions of verapamil with other cardiac drugs can potentiate both good and adverse effects. It has antagonistic effects with:

Oral anticoagulants
Salicylates
Sulfonamides

DISOPYRAMIDE

Another antiarrhythmic, disopyramide (Norpace), is a synthetic agent that decreases myocardial excitability, inhibits conduction, and may depress myocardial contractility.

Side effects can include:

Hypotension, dizziness, and chest pain
Edema and weight gain
Anticholinergic effects, including dry mouth, blurred vision, constipation, and urinary retention
Nausea, vomiting, bloating, and gas

Contraindications or extreme caution applies to:

History of angle-closure glaucoma
Heart block and congestive heart failure
Hepatic and renal disorders
Children, pregnancy, and lactation

Interactions of disopyramide occur with potentiation of the effects of:

Other cardiac drugs
Oral anticoagulants

LIDOCAINE

Local anesthetics (e.g., lidocaine) are administered for their antiarrhythmic effects.

Side effects are usually of short duration and dose related and can include:

CNS symptoms, including tremors, seizures, confusion, and blurred vision
Hypotension, bradycardia, and heart block
Respiratory arrest
ECG monitoring and availability of resuscitative equipment are necessary during IV administration of lidocaine.

Contraindications or extreme caution applies to:

Patients hypersensitive to local anesthetics of this type
Heart block and respiratory depression
Pregnancy

Interactions with other cardiac drugs may be additive or antagonistic and may potentiate adverse effects. Cimetidine may potentiate effects.

PROCAINAMIDE

Procainamide (Pronestyl) is usually administered orally in antiarrhythmic therapy. It is used primarily as prophylactic therapy to maintain normal rhythm after conversion by other methods. Its action is similar to that of quinidine.

Side effects are numerous and can include:

Hypotension
Tachycardia and conduction defects
Hypersensitivity reactions, including rash, fever, and weakness
Blood dyscracias, especially eosinophilia and leukopenia
Nausea and vomiting with overdose

Contraindications include:

Heart block and congestive heart failure
Hypersensitivity to local anesthetics of this type
Myasthenia gravis
Pregnancy

Interactions may occur with potentiation of:

Muscle relaxants
Anticholinergics
Other cardiac drugs

QUINIDINE

Quinidine (Quinaglute, Cardioquin) is one of the oldest antiarrhythmic agents. It acts by decreasing myocardial excitability and may depress myocardial contractility. Quinidine, like procainamide, is used primarily as prophylactic therapy to maintain normal rhythm after conversion by other methods. It is commonly administered orally in tablets or timed-release capsules.

Side effects are numerous and may necessitate cessation of treatment. They may include:

Tachycardia and syncope
Severe hypotension
Vascular collapse and respiratory arrest
Headache, tinnitus, vertigo, fever, and tremor
Confusion and apprehension
Vision abnormalities
Blood dyscracias, including anemia, clotting deficiencies, and leukopenia
Hepatic disorders
Precipitation of asthmatic attacks

Contraindications or extreme caution applies to:

Atrioventricular block and conduction defects
Electrolyte imbalance
Digitalis intoxication
Congestive heart failure and hypotension
Myasthenia gravis
Asthma and other respiratory disorders
Hyperthyroidism
Children, pregnancy, and lactation

Interactions with increased possibility of quinidine toxicity may occur with:

Muscle relaxants
Anticholinergics
Thiazide diuretics
Antacids or sodium bicarbonate
Anticonvulsants (e.g., phenytoin and phenobarbital)
Other cardiac drugs, especially digitalis and antihypertensives
Anticoagulants, whose action can be potentiated by quinidine

PHENYTOIN

Phenytoin (Dilantin) is most commonly administered as an anticonvulsant. However, it has been found to be useful in treating some arrhythmias not responsive to other antiarrhythmics or cardioversion. Phenytoin, administered IV, is considered the drug of choice in the treatment of arrhythmias caused by digitalis intoxication.

Side effects, common to antiarrhythmics, may include hypotension and bradycardia.

TABLE 25.1. CARDIAC GLYCOSIDES AND ANTIARRHYTHMICS

Generic Name	Trade Name	Dosage	Action
Cardiac Glycosides			
digoxin	Lanoxin	PO, IM, IV; dosage varies	Intermediate duration
digitoxin	Crystodigin	PO, IV; dosage varies	Prolonged duration
deslanoside	Cedilanid-D	IV 0.8–1.6 mg in divided doses	Rapid for emergencies
Antiarrhythmics			
propranolol[a,b]	Inderal	10–30 mg PO qid 0.5–3 mg IV	
verapamil[a,c]	Isoptin	5–10 mg IV, repeat if necessary in 30 min	
disopyramide	Norpace	150 mg PO q6h	
lidocaine	Xylocaine		
procainamide	Pronestyl	500 mg–1 g q4–6h IV or IM for emergency	
quinidine	Quinaglute, Cardioquin		
phenytoin	Dilantin		

[a]Has other cardiac uses.
[b]Beta-adrenergic blocker.
[c]Calcium blocker.

Contraindications or extreme caution applies to:

Heart block, congestive heart failure, and myocardial infarction
Respiratory depression
Pregnancy

PATIENT EDUCATION

Patients taking antiarrhythmics should be instructed regarding:

Immediate reporting of adverse side effects, especially palpitations, irregular or slow heartbeat, faintness, dizziness, weakness, respiratory distress, and visual disturbances
Holding medication, if there are side effects, until the physician is contacted
Rising slowly from reclining position
Modification of life-style to reduce stress
Mild exercise on a regular basis as approved by the physician
Not discontinuing medicine, even if the patient feels well
Taking proper dosage of medication on time, as prescribed, without skipping any dose
If medication is forgotten, *not* doubling the dose
Taking medication with a full glass of water, on an empty stomach, 1 h before or 2 h after meals, so that it will be absorbed more efficiently (unless stomach upset occurs or the physician prescribes otherwise)
Avoiding taking any other medication, including OTC medicines, unless approved by the physician

---

See Table 25.1 for a summary of the cardiac glycosides and antiarrhythmics.

Antihypertensives

Antihypertensives (hypotensives) are numerous in the treatment and management of all degrees of hypertension. In cases of mild hypertension, the initial treatment regimen usually includes diet modification (low salt or low sodium), weight reduction when indicated, mild exercise program (e.g., walking or swimming), curtailment of smoking, and stress reduction planning. In addition, the thiazide diuretics (see Chapter 15) are frequently prescribed to prevent sodium retention and edema, and for their hypotensive (blood pressure–lowering) effects. Antihypertensive drugs do *not* cure hypertension; they only control it. After withdrawal of the drug, the blood pressure will return to levels similar to those before treatment with medication, if all other factors remain the same. If antihypertensive therapy is to be terminated for some reason, the dosage should be gradually reduced, as abrupt withdrawal can cause rebound hypertension.

Drugs given to lower blood pressure act in various ways. The drug of choice varies according to the degree of hypertension (mild, moderate, or severe), other physical factors (especially other cardiac or renal complications), and effectiveness in individual cases. Frequently, antihypertensives are prescribed on a trial basis and then the dosage or medication is changed, and sometimes antihypertensives are combined for greater effectiveness and to reduce side effects. The health care worker must be observant of vital signs and side effects in order to assist the physician in the most effective treatment of hypertension on an individual basis.

Thiazide diuretics (see Chapter 15) are sometimes used alone to treat mild hypertension. Thiazides are also frequently combined with other antihypertensives to potentiate the hypotensive effects.

Side effects of antihypertensives are common, and the health care worker must be observant of changes in vital signs and adverse side effects. The most common side effect of the antihypertensives is *hypotension*, especially postural hypotension. Another side effect common to many of the antihypertensives is *bradycardia*. Exceptions include hydralazine (Apresoline), which can cause *tachycardia*.

RAUWOLFIA ALKALOIDS

Rauwolfia alkaloids, especially reserpine, are among the oldest medications used for hypotensive effect, and they possess a tranquilizing effect as well. The decrease in blood pressure is more gradual and frequently is associated with bradycardia. Fluid retention may accompany prolonged use unless diuretics are also prescribed. Sometimes rauwolfia alkaloids are combined with other antihypertensive drugs in order to reduce the dosage of each drug and minimize side effects.

Side effects (usually beginning with the letter *S*) can include:

Slower and safer action, with gradual blood pressure decrease and less hypotension

Sedative effect, with sleepiness and mental depression

Sexual dysfunction

Stomach ache (increased GI motility and increased gastric acid secretion may precipitate peptic ulcer symptoms or nausea, vomiting, and diarrhea)

Secretions increased in respiratory tract, leading to congestion

Bradycardia

Depression

Contraindications or extreme caution applies to:

History of peptic ulcer or ulcerative colitis

Activities requiring mental alertness (e.g., operating machinery or driving motor vehicles)

History of mental depression (can lead to suicide)

Epilepsy

Renal dysfunction

Pregnancy and lactation

Interactions may occur with:

Other antihypertensives and diuretics, which potentiate hypotensive action

Other cardiac drugs, especially digitalis, which may predispose patient to cardiac arrhythmias

MAO inhibitors, which can cause hypertension and excitation

Levodopa, with which antagonistic action of rauwolfia alkaloids may reduce effectiveness of L-dopa

---

PATIENT EDUCATION

Patients taking rauwolfia alkaloids should be instructed regarding:

Sedative side effects (taking care with tasks requiring alertness)

Reporting immediately to the physician any signs of mental depression, insomnia, or nightmares

Keeping medication in airtight, light-resistant container

Taking medication with meals as directed to reduce chance of stomach distress and reporting any GI symptoms to the physician at once

Not taking decongestants if nasal congestion occurs

Not taking any other medications or alcohol without consulting the physician first

Reporting to the physician at once any signs of slow or irregular heartbeat

Not discontinuing medication without consulting the physician

---

BETA-ADRENERGIC AND CALCIUM BLOCKERS

There are numerous other antihypertensives, and they vary in action. Included are beta-adrenergic blockers, such as propranolol (Inderal) and atenolol (Tenormin), and calcium blockers, such as diltiazem (Cardizem) (see "Antiarrhythmic Agents" for information on side effects, etc.).

METHYLDOPA

Another antihypertensive used for moderate to severe hypertension is methyldopa (Alodomet). It is usually administered with a diuretic.

Side effects, in addition to hypotension and drowsiness, can include:

Anemia or leukopenia
GI symptoms, including nausea, vomiting, diarrhea, constipation, and sore tongue
Sexual dysfunction
Liver disorders
Nasal congestion

Contraindications or extreme caution applies to:

Liver disorders
Dialysis patients
Blood dyscracias

Interactions may occur with:

Levodopa (can cause CNS effects and psychosis)
Lithium

HYDRALAZINE

Hydralazine (Apresoline) is frequently used in the treatment of moderate to severe hypertension, especially in patients with congestive heart failure, because it *increases* heart rate and cardiac output. The drug is generally used in conjunction with a diuretic and another hypotensive agent.

Side effects can include:

Tachycardia and palpitations
Headache and flushing
Orthostatic hypotension
GI effects, including nausea, vomiting, diarrhea, and constipation
Blood abnormalities
Allergic reactions (e.g., asthma)

Contraindications include pregnancy.

See Table 25.2 for a summary of the antihypertensives.

TABLE 25.2. ANTIHYPERTENSIVES

Generic Name	Trade Name	Dosage
Rauwolfia alkaloids		
reserpine	Serpasil	0.1–0.5 mg qd
Beta-Adrenergic Blockers		
propranolol	Inderal	10–30 mg PO qid
		0.5–3 mg IV
atenolol	Tenormin	50–100 mg PO qd
Calcium Blockers		
diltiazem	Cardizem	60 mg tid
Other Antihypertensives		
methyldopa	Aldomet	250–500 mg PO bid
clonidine	Catapres	0.1–0.8 mg PO
prazosin	Minipress	1.0–20 mg PO qd
hydralazine	Apresoline	10–50 mg qid

Note: This is only a representative list of the most commonly used drugs in this category. There are others.

PATIENT EDUCATION

For all antihypertensives, patients should be instructed regarding:

Immediate reporting of any adverse side effects, especially slow or irregular heartbeat, dizziness, weakness, breathing difficulty, gastric distress, and numbness or swelling of extremities

Taking medication on time as prescribed by the physician; *not* skipping a dose or doubling a dose; *not* discontinuing the medicine, even if the patient is feeling well, without consulting the physician first.

Rising slowly from reclining position to reduce lightheaded feeling

Taking care in driving a car or operating machinery if medication causes drowsiness (ask the physician, nurse, or pharmacist about the specific medication, since medicines differ and individual reactions differ; older people are more susceptible to this effect)

Potentiation of adverse side effects by alcohol, especially dizziness, weakness, sleepiness, and confusion

Reduction of smoking to help lower blood pressure

Importance of diet in control of blood pressure; following the physician's instructions regarding appropriate diet for the individual, which may include a low-salt or -sodium or weight-reduction diet if indicated

Avoiding hot tubs and hot showers, which may cause weakness or fainting

Mild exercise, on a regular basis, as approved by the physician

Coronary Vasodilators

Coronary vasodilators are used in the treatment of angina. When there is insufficient blood supply (ischemia) to a part, the result is acute pain. The most common form of angina is angina pectoris, chest pain resulting from decreased blood supply to the heart muscle. Obstruction or constriction of the coronary arteries results in angina pectoris. Vasodilators are administered to dilate these blood vessels and stop attacks of angina or reduce the frequency of angina when administered prophylactically.

Coronary vasodilators used in the treatment and prophylactic management of angina include nitrates, beta blockers, and calcium blockers.

The nitrates used most commonly for relief of acute angina pectoris, as well as for long-term prophylactic management, are nitroglycerin and isosorbide (Isordil, Sorbitrate).

Nitroglycerin is available in several forms and can be administered in sublingual tablets allowed to dissolve under the tongue or intrabuccal tablets allowed to dissolve in the cheek pouch for relief of acute angina pectoris. If relief is not attained after a single dose during an acute attack, additional tablets may be administered at 5-min intervals, with *no more than three doses given in a 15-min period*. If chest pain is not relieved after three doses, a physician should be contacted at once because unrelieved chest pain can indicate acute myocardial infarction.

Nitroglycerin is also available in timed-release capsules and tablets, and in a solution that must be diluted carefully according to the manufacturer's instructions for IV administration. Nitroglycerin tablets and capsules must be stored only in glass containers with tightly fitting metal screw tops away from heat. Plastic containers can absorb the medication, and air, heat, or moisture can cause loss of potency. Impaired potency of the SL tablets can be detected by the patient if there is an absence of the tingling sensation under the tongue common to this form of administration.

For long-term prophylactic management of angina pectoris, nitroglycerin is frequently applied topically as a transdermal system. One type of nitroglycerin that is absorbed through the skin is Nitrol ointment, applied with an applicator-measuring (Appliruler) paper. Usual dosage is 0.5–2 inches applied every 4–6 h. The ointment is spread lightly (not massaged or rubbed) over any nonhairy skin area, and the applicator paper is taped in place. Care must be taken to avoid touching the ointment when applying (accidental absorption through the skin of the fingers can cause headache). If nitroglycerin ointment is discontinued, the dose and frequency must be decreased gradually to prevent sudden withdrawal reactions.

Another topical nitroglycerin product, which has longer action, is in patch form (e.g., Nitro-Dur or Transderm-Nitro). The skin patch is applied every 24 h to clean, dry, hairless areas of the upper arm or body. Do not apply below the elbow or knee. The sites should be rotated to avoid skin irritation and raw, scarred, or callused areas should be avoided. Dosage varies widely, from 2.5-mg–15-mg patches. Check prescribed dosage carefully.

Another nitrate used for acute relief of angina pectoris and for prophylactic long-term management is isosorbide. It is available in sublingual, PO, or chewable tablets and in timed-release capsules.

Side effects of the nitrates can include:

Headache (usually diminishes over time)
Postural hypotension, including dizziness, weakness, and syncope (patients should be sitting during administration of fast-acting nitrates)
Transient flushing
Blurred vision and dry mouth (discontinue drug with these symptoms)
Hypersensitivity reactions, enhanced by alcohol, including nausea, vomiting, diarrhea, cold sweats, tachycardia, and syncope

Contraindications or extreme caution applies to:

Glaucoma
GI hypermotility or malabsorption (with timed-release forms)
Intracranial pressure
Severe anemia
Hypotension

PATIENT EDUCATION

Patients receiving coronary vasodilators (nitrates) should be instructed regarding:

Administering fast-acting tablets (sublingual or buccal) while sitting down because the patient may become lightheaded
Rising slowly from a reclining position
Not drinking alcohol while taking these medicines, which can cause serious drop in blood pressure
Using timed-release capsules or tablets to prevent attacks (they work too slowly to help once an attack has started)
Taking timed-release capsules or tablets on an empty stomach with a full glass of water
Allowing sublingual tablets to dissolve under the tongue or in the cheek pouch and not chewing or swallowing them
Chewing chewable tablets thoroughly and holding them in the mouth for 2 min without any food or water in the mouth
Repeating sublingual, buccal, or chewable tablets in 5–10 min for a maximum of three tablets (if no relief of chest pain within 15–30 min, call the physician at once)
Not discontinuing medication suddenly if administered for several weeks (dosage must be reduced gradually under physician's supervision)
Sensations to be expected, including facial flushing, headache for a short time, lightheadedness upon rising too suddenly (if these symptoms persist or become more severe, or other symptoms, such as irregular heartbeat or blurred vision, occur, notify the physician at once)
Preventing attacks of angina by administering a sublingual or chewable tablet before physical exertion or emotional stress (it is preferable to avoid physical or emotional stress when possible)

Interactions of nitrates may occur with alcohol, which potentiates hypotensive effects.

For long-term prophylactic treatment of angina pectoris, beta blockers, such as propranolol (Inderal), and calcium blockers, such as nifedipine (Procardia) and verapamil (Isoptin), are frequently used (see "Antiarrhythmic Agents" for information on side effects, etc.).

Peripheral Vasodilators

Peripheral vasodilators, such as tolazoline (Priscoline), are used as an adjunctive treatment in vasospastic disorders associated with arteriosclerosis, diabetic arteriosclerosis, gangrene, scleroderma, Buerger's disease, Raynaud's disease, frostbite, or thrombophlebitis.

Side effects of tolazoline include:

Increased secretions (saliva, gastric, sweat, and tears)
Tachycardia, cardiac arrhythmias, angina, hypertension, and paradoxical hypotension
Blood dyscrasias
Headache and dizziness

Contraindications or extreme caution applies to:

Gastritis and peptic ulcer
Coronary artery disease and cerebrovascular accident

Interactions may occur with:

Alcohol, with possible severe disulfiram-like reaction (see Chapter 20)
Epinephrine, which may cause fall in blood pressure followed by exaggerated rebound hypertension

Vasoconstrictors

Vasoconstrictors are adrenergic in action (see Chapter 18). Drugs such as norepinephrine (Levophed) or metaraminol bitartrate (Aramine) constrict blood vessels, resulting in increased systolic and diastolic blood pressure. These drugs are used mainly in the treatment of shock.

Side effects can include:

Headache (may be a symptom of hypertension)
Weakness, dizziness, tremor, and pallor

Respiratory difficulty or apnea
Pain in the cardiac area
Palpitation, bradycardia, cardiac arrhythmias
Necrosis of tissues

Cautions include:

Close monitoring of IV site
Close monitoring of blood pressure and other vital signs

Anticoagulants

Anticoagulants are divided into two groups: coumarin derivatives and heparin. The action of these two classes is quite different. However, their purpose is the same: to prevent formation of clots or decrease the extension of existing clots in such conditions as venous thrombosis, pulmonary embolism, and coronary occlusion. The coumarin derivatives and heparin do *not* dissolve clots; they only interfere with the coagulation process as a prophylaxis.

COUMARIN DERIVATIVES

Coumarin derivatives (e.g., warfarin) are administered *orally*. The coumarin derivatives alter the synthesis of blood coagulation factors in the liver by interfering with the action of vitamin K. The *antidote* for serious bleeding complications during coumarin therapy is *vitamin K*. The action of the coumarin derivatives is slower than that of heparin, and therefore these drugs are generally used as follow-up for long-term anticoagulant therapy. Measurement of the prothrombin time (PT) is the most commonly used laboratory method of monitoring therapy with coumarin derivatives. The PT serves as a guide in determining dosage.

Interactions of coumarin derivatives with many drugs have been reported. Concurrent administration of any other drug should be investigated, and the following drugs should be *avoided* if possible. Some of the drugs that may *increase* response to coumarin derivatives include:

Anabolic steroids
Chloral hydrate and alcohol (acute intoxication)
Disulfiram
All NSAID, including aspirin
Tricyclic antidepressants
Thyroid drugs
Thiazides and quinidine

Some of the drugs that may *decrease* response to coumarin derivatives include:

Alcohol (chronic alcoholism)
Barbiturates
Estrogen (including oral contraceptives)
Corticosteroids

HEPARIN

Heparin is not absorbed from the GI tract and must be administered *intravenously* or *subcutaneously*. Heparin acts on thrombin, inhibiting the action of fibrin in clot formation. The *antidote* for serious bleeding complications during heparin therapy is *protamine sulfate*. When administered IV, the action of heparin is immediate. A *dilute* solution of heparin is also used to maintain patency of indwelling intravenous catheters and adapters used for intermittent IV therapy. Measurement of the activated partial thromboplastic time (APTT) is the most common laboratory test for monitoring heparin therapy. When long-term anticoagulant therapy is begun with coumarin derivatives, there is a short-term overlap period in which both heparin and coumarin derivatives are administered concurrently.

Side effects of all anticoagulants can include:

Major hemorrhage
Minor bleeding (e.g., petechiae, nosebleed, and bruising)
Blood in urine (hematuria) or stools (melena)

Contraindications of anticoagulants include:

GI disorders and ulceration of GI tract
Hepatic and renal dysfunction
Blood dyscrasias
Preoperative administration
Pregnancy, especially third trimester

See Table 25.3 for a summary of the coronary and peripheral vasodilators and the anticoagulants.

TABLE 25.3. CORONARY VASODILATORS, PERIPHERAL VASODILATORS, AND ANTICOAGULANTS

Generic Name	Trade Name	Dosage
Coronary Vasodilators[a]		
Nitrates		
nitroglycerin	Nitroglycerin	
	tabs	SL 1–3 tabs q5min × 3 maximum in 15 min
	tabs	Buccal 1–3 tabs q5min × 3 maximum in 15 min
	caps or tabs	Timed-release 1.3–9 mg q8–12h
	Nitrol ointment 2%	1–2 inches q4–6h, rotate site
	Transderm-Nitro, Nitro-Dur patches	1 qd, rotate site
isosorbide	Isordil, Sorbitrate	SL, or chewable tabs, 2.5–10 mg × 3 maximum in 30 min
		Prophylactic, 10–20 mg tid or qid ac
		Timed-release 40–80 mg q6–12h
Peripheral Vasodilator		
tolazoline	Priscoline	IV, IM, SC; dosage varies
Anticoagulants		
warfarin	Coumadin	Caps or tabs PO; dosage varies
heparin	Heparin	IV, SC; dosage varies

[a]For prevention and treatment of angina pectoris.
Note: Beta blockers and calcium blockers are also administered prophylactically for angina pectoris, and can be given concurrently with the nitrates.

PATIENT EDUCATION

It is *very important* that patients on anticoagulant therapy be instructed regarding:

Careful daily observation of skin, gums, urine, and stools, and *immediate* reporting of any signs of bleeding

Avoiding sports and activities that may cause bleeding

Immediate reporting to the physician of any falls, blows, or injuries (internal bleeding is always a possibility)

Special care with shaving (electric razor only) and with teeth brushing or dental floss

Wearing an identification tag or carrying a card indicating use of anticoagulant

Immediate reporting of severe or continued headache or backache, dizziness, joint pain or swelling, tarry stools, abdominal distention, and vomiting of material resembling coffee grounds

Avoiding any other medication without the physician's approval, especially OTC aspirin, anti-inflammatory drugs, and antacids

Avoiding alcohol

Cardiovascular Drugs

Note the drugs listed according to category and complete all columns. Learn generic or trade names as specified by instructor.

CLASSIFICATIONS AND DRUGS	PURPOSE	SIDE EFFECTS	CONTRAINDICATIONS OR CAUTIONS	PATIENT EDUCATION
Cardiac Glycosides				
1. digoxin				
2. digitoxin				
3. deslanoside				
Antiarrhythmics				
1. propranolol (a beta-adrenergic blocker with other uses)				
2. verapamil (a calcium blocker with other uses)				
3. lidocaine				
4. procainamide				
5. quinidine				
6. phenytoin				
Antihypertensives				
1. reserpine				
2. methyldopa				
3. prazosin				
4. hydralazine				

CLASSIFICATIONS AND DRUGS	PURPOSE	SIDE EFFECTS	CONTRAINDICATIONS OR CAUTIONS	PATIENT EDUCATION
Vasodilators				

1. nitroglycerin
   Tabs SL
   Ointment
   Patch				

2. isosorbide				
Anticoagulants				
1. dicumarol				
2. heparin				

26

Respiratory System Drugs

OBJECTIVES

Upon completion of this chapter, the student will be able to:

1. Describe uses of and precautions necessary with oxygen therapy.
2. Explain the purpose of carbon dioxide inhalations.
3. Define bronchodilator, mucolytic, expectorant, and antitussive.
4. Classify a list of respiratory system drugs according to action.
5. List uses, side effects, and contraindications for bronchodilators and antitussives.
6. Explain appropriate patient education for those receiving respiratory system drugs.

Therapeutic measures for respiratory distress include oxygen, respiratory stimulants, bronchodilators, mucolytics, expectorants, and antitussives.

Oxygen

Oxygen is used therapeutically for hypoxia (insufficient oxygen). Some of the conditions for which oxygen is indicated are heart and lung diseases, carbon monoxide poisoning, and some central nervous conditions with respiratory difficulty or failure. Oxygen may be administered by endotracheal intubation, nasal catheter or cannula, masks, tents, and hoods.

Side effects of oxygen delivered at too high a percentage for prolonged periods of time can include:

Hypoventilation (apnea), particularly with COPD
Acidosis
Confusion
Visual disturbances
Blindness (in premature infants)

Precautions include:

Patients with COPD (O_2 rate cannot be too high, which may cause apnea)
Danger of fire when oxygen is used; smoking, matches, and electrical equipment that may spark (e.g., electric razors, hair dryers) not allowed in rooms where oxygen is in use

Respiratory Stimulants

Respiratory stimulants include:

Caffeine and sodium benzoate administered parenterally in the treatment of apnea in the newborn, alcoholic stupor, and occasionally in drug overdose (see Chapter 20)
Carbon dioxide inhalations to increase both depth and rate of respiration (e.g., in treatment of hyperventilation or hiccups)

Bronchodilators

Bronchodilators (adrenergic in action) are used to relax the smooth muscles in the respiratory tract and reverse bronchospasm, relieving dyspnea and wheezing and improving pulmonary function. Treatment of chronic obstructive pulmonary disease includes such conditions as asthma, chronic bronchitis, and emphysema. The most commonly used bronchodilators are *theophylline* compounds (e.g., Aminophyllin), which are available in various forms (e.g., tablets, extended-release capsules, rectal suppositories, and IV solutions). Theophyllines are also available in combinations with adrenergics, sedatives, and expectorants, which should be used with care because of possible potentiation of adverse effects. One such combination is Tedral, which combines theophylline with an adrenergic agent (ephedrine) and a sedative (phenobarbital). Such combinations should only be used on a short-term, intermittent basis when insomnia is a problem. Theophylline is usually administered in single-ingredient preparations because of greater safety and to facilitate dosage adjustments.

Side effects can include:

GI distress: nausea, vomiting, abdominal pain, anorexia
CNS stimulation: nervousness, insomnia, irritability (in children can progress to convulsions)
Cardiac effects: palpitation, tachycardia, arrhythmias
Urinary frequency (mild diuresis)
Hyperglycemia

Caution applies to:

Rapid IV injection which can cause dizziness, cardiac arrhythmias, or cardiac arrest
IM injection of aminophyllin, *contraindicated* because it can produce pain and sloughing of tissues
Suppositories, which can cause rectal irritation
Toxicity, which is more prominent in children, elderly and those with cardiovascular, kidney, or liver dysfunction, and patients with diabetes, peptic ulcer, or glaucoma
Theophylline blood levels, which should be monitored with large doses and/ or long-term use

Interactions occur with:

Digitalis or other cardiac drugs, which may increase potential for toxicity
Oral anticoagulant action increased
Cimetidine, allopurinol, propranolol, and erythromycin, which increase theophylline levels

TABLE 26.1. BRONCHODILATORS

Generic Name	Trade Name	Dosage	Comments
theophylline compound (xanthine derivative)	Aminophyllin	PO 600–1,600 mg qd in divided doses	Possible GI distress, irritation
		500 mg supp bid or qd	Possible rectal irritation
		IV 0.3–0.9 mg/kg of body weight	Inject IV slowly
	Elixophyllin, Theodur	PO timed-release cap q12h	
theophylline combination of theophylline, ephedrine, and phenobarbital	Quibron	PO 150–300 mg q6–8h	Test blood sugar (may be elevated)
	Tedral	PO 1–2 tabs q6h	Useful with insomnia; intermittent use
terbutaline	Brethine	PO 2.5–5 mg tid	
	Brethaire	SC 0.25 mg, repeat 15–30 min PRN	
isoproterenol	Isuprel	SL 10–15 mg, nebulizer 1 : 100–1 : 200	Related to epinephrine; caution with diabetes; blood sugar elevation possible
bitolterol	Tornalate	Aerosol inhalations q8h PRN	

Sympathomimetics (*adrenergics*), for example, epinephrine SC or isoproterenol (Isuprel) by nebulizer or sublingual, are sometimes given at the same time as theophylline. Metaproterenol (Alupent) and terbutaline also have adrenergic action.

Side effects of the adrenergics include potentiation of theophylline effects with increased risk of toxicity especially:

CNS stimulation
Cardiac irregularities

See Chapter 18 for additional information regarding bronchodilators (adrenergics).
See Table 26.1 for a summary of the bronchodilators.

Mucolytics and Expectorants

Mucolytics, for example, Mucomyst, liquify pulmonary secretions. Expectorants, (out of the chest), for example, guaifenesin, increase secretions, reduce viscosity, and help expel sputum. Adequate fluid intake also helps loosen and liquify secretions. Cough syrups commonly combine various expectorants in the symptomatic management of coughs associated with upper respiratory infections, bronchitis, sinusitis, and COPD.

TABLE 26.2. MUCOLYTICS AND EXPECTORANTS

Generic Name	Trade Name	Dosage	Comments
acetylcysteine	Mucomyst	q2–6h	Used with nebulizer or IPPB
guaifenesin	Robitussin	PO 100–200 mg (1–2 tsp) q3–4h	
terpin hydrate		PO 5–10 ml q3–4h	

Side effects can include:

Nausea and vomiting
Stomatitis
Runny nose
Drowsiness

Contraindications or caution applies to:

Some asthmatics (prone to bronchospasm)
Cardiovascular disease and hypertension
Diabetes
Hyperthyroidism

See Table 26.2 for a summary of the mucolytics and expectorants.

Antitussives

Antitussives are medications to prevent coughing in patients not requiring a productive cough. Coughing, a reflex mechanism, helps eliminate secretions from the respiratory tract. A dry, nonproductive cough can cause fatigue, insomnia, and in some cases pain to the patient (e.g., pleurisy and fractured ribs). Narcotic antitussives may be used to relieve these patients but have limited use because of respiratory depressant action and bronchial constriction (e.g., morphine). Codeine, a narcotic with fewer side effects, is frequently used, but is addictive with long-term use. Codeine is added to some cough syrups.

Side effects of narcotic antitussives can include:

Respiratory depression
Constipation
Urinary retention
Sedation and dizziness
Nausea and vomiting

TABLE 26.3. ANTITUSSIVES

Generic Name	Trade Name	Dosage	Comments
Narcotic			
codeine	Many combinations	Dosage varies; frequently	Not for extended use; can develop
hydrocodone	in cough syrups	5mg/5ml q4–6h	tolerance and physical
			dependence; watch for side effects
Nonnarcotic			
dextromethorphan	Romilar	20–30 mg q4–6h,	No analgesic properties
		lozenges or syrup	
diphenhydramine	Benylin	2 tsp q4h	
benzonatate	Tessalon	100–200 mg tid	

Contraindications include:

Addiction-prone patients
Asthma
COPD

Nonnarcotic antitussives (e.g., dextromethorphan) are more frequently used because they do not depress respirations, do not cause addiction, and have few side effects.

Contraindications include:

Asthma
COPD

See Table 26.3 for a summary of the antitussives.

PATIENT EDUCATION

Patients taking respiratory system drugs should be instructed regarding:

Care in taking medications only as prescribed and required
Avoid combining respiratory system drugs with other prescription or OTC drugs or alcohol, which could potentiate CNS stimulation or depression resulting in serious adverse side effects
Avoiding self-medication when cardiac, thyroid, or CNS conditions are present
Liberal intake of fluids, which is encouraged to help liquify secretions
Benefit from desensitization therapy and air-conditioned environmental control for patients with allergic conditions
Avoiding air pollution (e.g., smoke-filled rooms)
Exercises (e.g., swimming) that increase lung capacity and help reduce the necessity for medication

---

WORKSHEET FOR CHAPTER 26

Respiratory Drugs

Note the drugs listed according to category and complete all columns. Learn generic or trade names as specified by instructor.

CLASSIFICATIONS AND DRUGS	PURPOSE	SIDE EFFECTS	CONTRAINDICATIONS OR CAUTIONS	PATIENT EDUCATION
Bronchodilators				
1. Aminophyllin				
2. Theodur				
3. Tedral				
4. Isuprel				
Mucolytics and Expectorants				
1. Mucomyst				
2. Robitussin				
Antitussives				
1. codeine				
2. Romilar				
3. Benylin				

27

Antihistamines, Preoperative Medications, and Local Anesthetics

OBJECTIVES

Upon completion of this chapter, the student will be able to:

1. Describe the action and uses of the antihistamines.
2. List the side effects, contraindications, and interactions of the antihistamines.
3. List the three most common components of preoperative injections and give examples of each.
4. Describe side effects and cautions with preoperative medications.
5. Identify two medications that are incompatible with others in the same syringe.
6. Differentiate the five methods of administration of local anesthetics.
7. Describe side effects and cautions with local anesthetics.
8. Explain the interactions of epinephrine with local anesthetic.
9. List the important aspects of patient education with antihistamines and preoperatives and local anesthetics.

Antihistamines

Antihistamines, such as diphenhydramine (Benadryl), competitively antagonize the histamine$_1$ receptor sites. Through this action, the antihistamines combat the increased capillary permeability and edema, inflammation, and itch caused by sudden histamine release.

Antihistamines are not curative, but provide *symptomatic relief of allergic symptoms* caused by histamine release. They are also used as adjunctive treatment of anaphylactic reactions *after* the acute symptoms (e.g., laryngeal edema and shock) have been controlled with epinephrine and corticosteroids.

Antihistamines are used to treat the symptoms of allergies (e.g., rhinitis, conjunctivitis, and rash). However, when antihistamines are used to reduce nasal secretions in the common cold, the consequent thickening of bronchial secretions may result in further airway obstruction, especially in those with chronic obstructive pulmonary disease (COPD) and asthma.

Some antihistamines are used in the symptomatic treatment of vertigo associated with pathology of the middle ear or in the prevention and treatment of motion sickness (see Chapter 16).

Side effects of the antihistamines are anticholinergic in action and include:

Drying of secretions, especially of the eyes, ears, nose, and throat
Sedation, dizziness, and hypotension, especially in the elderly
Muscular weakness and decreased coordination
Urinary retention and constipation
Visual disorders
Paradoxical excitement, insomnia, and tremors, especially in children

Contraindications or extreme caution applies to:

COPD and asthma
Persons operating machinery or driving a car
Elderly patients
Cardiovascular disorders
Benign prostatic hypertrophy (BPH)
Infants, pregnancy, and lactation

PATIENT EDUCATION

Patients should be instructed regarding:

Avoiding frequent or prolonged use of antihistamines, which may cause increased bronchial or nasal congestion and dry cough
No self-medication (check with the physician first) in those with COPD or cardiovascular disorders, BPH, the elderly, and children
Caution with those operating machinery becasue of sedative effect
No mixing with alcohol or any other CNS depressant drugs

TABLE 27.1. ANTIHISTAMINES

Generic Name	Trade Name	Dosage
brompheniramine	Dimetane	4 mg q4–6h sol, tabs, extended-release tabs 10 mg q6–12h IM or IV
diphenhydramine	Benadryl	25–50 mg PO q4–6h 10–50 mg IM or IV q4–6h
chlorpheniramine	Chlor-Trimeton	4 mg q4–6h
promethazine HCl	Phenergan	Varies with condition and use as preoperative medication or antiemetic (see Chapter 16)
hydroxyzine	Vistaril	25–100 mg deep IM or Z-track, preoperative medication or tranquilizer, also PO

Interactions may occur with:

Potentiation of CNS depression with tranquilizers, analgesics, hypnotics, alcohol, and muscle relaxants

Potentiation of anticholinergic effect with MAO inhibitors

Phenothiazine antihistamines, which antagonize the vasopressor effect of epinephrine

See Table 27.1 for a summary of the antihistamines.

Preoperative Medications

Preoperative medications, given before general anesthetics, commonly include a combination of an *anticholinergic* (antimuscarinic) with one or more of the following: sedative-hypnotic or tranquilizer, and/or opiate.

The *anticholinergics* (see Chapter 18) most commonly used as preoperative medications include atropine, glycopyrrolate (Robinul), and scopolamine. They reduce the secretions of the nose, mouth, pharynx, bronchi, and GI tract. In addition, atropine acts as a bronchodilator, and atropine and scopolamine reduce the incidence of laryngospasm. The anticholinergics also decrease gastric activity.

Side effects of the anticholinergic preoperative medications can include:

Drying of all secretions
Decreased GI and genitourinary motility, constipation, and urinary retention
Flushing
Cardiac arrhythmias and tachycardia
Confusion and/or excitement, especially with the elderly and infants
Hallucinations with scopolamine

TABLE 27.2. PREOPERATIVE ANTICHOLINERGICS

Generic Name	Trade Name	Dosage
atropine	Atropine	0.4–0.6 mg, SC, IM, IV
scopolamine	Scopolamine	0.3–0.6, SC, IM, IV
glycopyrrolate	Robinul	0.2 mg, SC, IM, IV

Contraindications or caution applies to:

COPD
Gastric ulcer and hiatal hernia
GI infections and ulcerative colitis
Angle-closure glaucoma
BPH and renal disorders
Myasthenia gravis
Cardiovascular disease
Elderly patients and infants

Interactions with potentiation of sedation occurs with CNS depressants.

PATIENT EDUCATION

Patients receiving anticholinergics should be instructed regarding side effects to expect (e.g., dry mouth, blurred vision, and sedation).

See Table 27.2 for a summary of the preoperative anticholinergics.

Sometimes hydroxyzine (Vistaril), an antihistamine, is given instead of the anticholinergic for its sedative, tranquilizing, antisecretory, antiemetic, and bronchodilating effects (see Table 27.1).

Commonly administered concurrently with the anticholinergics are *sedative-hypnotic barbiturates*, such as *pentobarbital* (*never combine in a syringe with any other medication*).

Another drug commonly included in preoperative injections is a narcotic, such as meperidine (Demerol) 50–100 mg IM. This may be combined in the same syringe with the anticholinergic to reduce the number of injections given concurrently.

Preoperative medications are usually administered intramuscularly 30–60 min before the start of anesthesia.

Light anesthesia for short-term surgical and diagnostic procedures is sometimes achieved by intravenous administration of diazepam (Valium) 10–20 mg (*never combined in a syringe with any other medication*).

PATIENT EDUCATION

Patients receiving preoperative medications should be instructed regarding:

Side effects to expect (e.g., dry mouth, blurred vision, sleepiness, weakness, and dizziness)
Remaining in bed after preoperative medication is given to prevent falls or injury

---

Local Anesthetics

Local anesthetics are administered topically to produce temporary loss of sensation or feeling in that specific area only. Local anesthetics may be administered by the following five methods:

1. *Infiltration anesthesia.* Achieved by injecting the local anesthetic solution into the skin, subcutaneous tissue, or mucous membranes of the area to be anesthetized. It is used in minor surgical and dental procedures (e.g., procaine or lidocaine).

2. *Direct topical anesthesia.* Achieved by application of the local anesthetic directly to the surface of the area to be anesthetized. It is used for temporary relief of painful eye, ear, nose, and throat or dental conditions or to reduce the discomfort of minor procedures (e.g., cocaine solution, *never* injected, is applied to nasal mucosa before nasal surgery; benzocaine lozenges or gels are for throat or mouth pain; benzocaine otic drops are for ear pain; Nupercaine ointment is for hemorrhoids, episiotomy, or minor skin lesions; or ethyl chloride spray is for very short surgical procedures such as incision and drainage of carbuncles.)

3. *Peripheral nerve block (regional anesthesia).* Achieved by injecting a local anesthetic solution into or around nerves or ganglia supplying the area to be anesthetized (e.g., face or extremities).

4. *Spinal anesthesia.* Achieved by injecting local anesthetic solutions intrathecally (into the subarachnoid space of the spinal canal) either in the lumbar region or lower (saddle block), depending on the area to be anesthetized. Spinal anesthesia is used for abdominal surgery or obstetrics.

5. *Epidural anesthesia.* Produced by injecting local anesthetic solution into the epidural space just outside the spinal cord, for example, caudal (sacral) anesthesia, frequently used in obstetrics.

Although local anesthetics do not produce loss of consciousness, there is some degree of systemic absorption. CNS and cardiovascular effects are possible, depending on the sensitivity of the individual and the amount and type of local anesthesia used. Epinephrine may be added to the local anesthetic solution to prolong the duration of action, and therefore adrenergic effects are possible (e.g., palpitations, tachycardia, and anxiety). Hypersensitivity reactions with anaphylaxis are possible, and therefore resuscitative procedures, drugs, and equipment should always be available when local anesthetics are administered. Obtaining a history of allergy before administration is essential.

Side effects can include:

Hypersensitivity reaction, edema, and anaphylaxis
Hypotension and cardiac arrest (*not* as likely when epinephrine is added)
Respiratory difficulties (especially with high spinals)
CNS depression or excitation and seizures

TABLE 27.3. LOCAL ANESTHETICS

Generic Name	Trade Name	Dosage
benzocaine	Chloraseptic, Americaine, Anbesol	Lozenges, sol
cocaine		Sol (never inject)
dibucaine	Nupercaine	Ointment, injection
ethyl chloride		Spray
lidocaine	Xylocaine[a]	0.5%, 1%, 1.5%, 2%, and higher with spinals
procaine	Novocain[a]	1% and 2% (higher with spinals)

[a]Available plain or in combination with epinephrine (very important to note difference).

Contraindications or extreme caution applies to:

Cardiovascular disease

Hyperthyroidism

Hepatic disorders

Pregnancy

History of allergy

Elderly patients

Interaction of local anesthetics with *epinephrine* not only prolongs the duration of the anesthesia but also helps localize the anesthesia, thus *decreasing* systemic effects.

PATIENT EDUCATION

Patients should be instructed regarding:

Accurate reporting of allergies or other physical conditions prior to local anesthetic

Prompt reporting of any side effects during local anesthesia (e.g., palpitations, nervousness, vertigo, and weakness)

Reassurance about the safety of the procedure both before and during the administration of local anesthetics

---

See Table 27.3 for a summary of the local anesthetics.

WORKSHEET FOR CHAPTER 27

Antihistamines, Preoperative Medications, and Local Anesthetics

Note the drugs listed according to category and complete all columns. Learn generic or trade names as specified by instructor.

CLASSIFICATIONS AND DRUGS	PURPOSE	SIDE EFFECTS	CONTRAINDICATIONS OR CAUTIONS	PATIENT EDUCATION
Antihistamines				
1. Dimetane				
2. Benadryl				
Preoperative Medications: Drying Agents				
1. atropine				
2. scopolamine				
3. Robinul				
4. Vistaril				
Preoperative Medications: Sedatives and Opiates				
1. pentobarbital				
2. meperidine				
3. diazepam (Valium)				
Local Anesthetics				
1. benzocaine				
2. cocaine				
3. ethyl chloride				
4. Xylocaine, Novocain				

COMPREHENSIVE REVIEW EXAM FOR PART II

1. Deficiency of potassium may result in:

   a. diarrhea
   b. petechiae

   c. cardiac arrhythmias
   d. GI bleeding

2. Which would be *least* likely to require vitamin or mineral supplements?

   a. executive secretary
   b. nursing mother

   c. adolescent
   d. alcoholic

3. The following statements are true of vitamin C *except:*

   a. destroyed by heat
   b. unstable with antacids

   c. found in citrus fruits
   d. prevents upper respiratory infection

4. Which condition will slow absorption of topical medication?

   a. heat
   b. moisture

   c. macerated skin
   d. callused skin

5. All of the following are antipruritics *except:*

   a. Benzocaine
   b. Caladryl

   c. Cuticura
   d. Cortaid

6. If a superinfection (e.g., diarrhea) occurs with antibiotic therapy, the patient should be told to do all of the following *except:*

   a. discontinue medication
   b. drink buttermilk

   c. eat yogurt
   d. try a bland diet

7. Most antibiotics are best administered:

   a. with fruit juice
   b. with antacids

   c. 1 h ac
   d. ½ h pc

8. Allergic hypersensitivity can be manifested in all of the following ways *except:*

   a. diarrhea
   b. rash

   c. hives
   d. anaphylaxis

9. Which of the following would be most likely to develop a penicillin reaction?

   a. premature infant
   b. cancer patient
   c. diabetic
   d. allergic asthmatic

10. The following statements are true of atropine *except:*

    a. used as a mydriatic
    b. used as a cycloplegic
    c. treatment for glaucoma
    d. can cause blurred vision

11. The following statements are true of corticosteroid ophthalmic ointment *except:*

    a. can delay healing
    b. used short term
    c. anti-inflammatory
    d. used for infections

12. Which statement is *not* true of Pyridium?

    a. has antibacterial action
    b. has local anesthetic effect
    c. turns urine red-orange
    d. has analgesic action

13. The following side effects are possible with thiazide diuretics *except:*

    a. hypokalemia
    b. hypoglycemia
    c. increased uric acid
    d. muscle weakness

14. The thiazides are used to treat all of the following conditions *except:*

    a. hypertension
    b. congestive heart failure
    c. gout
    d. edema

15. Which term does *not* describe a purpose for antineoplastic drugs?

    a. cytotoxic
    b. analeptic
    c. palliative
    d. remission

16. Which is *not* a frequent side effect of antineoplastic drugs?

    a. jaundice
    b. diarrhea
    c. ulcers of mucosa
    d. nausea and vomiting

17. Which side effect is *not* associated with atropine?

    a. diaphoresis
    b. confusion
    c. blurred vision
    d. urinary retention

18. Which side effect is *not* associated with epinephrine?

    a. hypertension
    b. hypoglycemia
    c. tachycardia
    d. tremor

19. Which is *not* an action of cholinergic drugs?

    a. increased peristalsis
    b. lowered intraocular pressure
    c. reduced salivation
    d. bladder contraction

20. Which dose of epinephrine is the *only* appropriate one?

    a. 0.2 ml IM   c. 1.5 ml IV
    b. 0.3 ml SC   d. 1.0 ml SC

Jim J. is admitted to the emergency room with a history of insecticide poisoning (cholinergic action). Questions 21 and 22 are related to Jim's situation:

21. Jim's symptoms might include all of the following *except:*

    a. facial flushing   c. diarrhea
    b. diaphoresis   d. nausea

22. His treatment would most likely include which drug?

    a. Prostigmin   c. Atropine
    b. Adrenalin   d. Isuprel

23. Which statement is *not* true of Lomotil?

    a. slows peristalsis   c. has drying effect
    b. contains atropine   d. used for food poisoning

24. Which laxative would be used for chronic constipation?

    a. milk of magnesia   c. Ex-Lax
    b. Dulcolax   d. Metamucil

25. Which medication is *not* an antimetic?

    a. Phenergan   c. Dramamine
    b. Imodium   d. Compazine

26. The most likely prescription for frequent gas pains is:

    a. milk of magnesia   c. Mylicon
    b. Colace   d. Metamucil

27. Which statement is *not* true of the nonsteroidal antiinflammatory drugs?

    a. alleviate pain of arthritis   c. used long term sometimes
    b. raise prostaglandin levels   d. reduce joint swelling

28. Which drug is *not* a muscle relaxant?

    a. Robaxin   c. Delalutin
    b. Valium   d. Flexeril

29. Which is *not* a possible side effect with narcotic use?

    a. constipation   c. urinary retention
    b. tachycardia   d. blurred vision

30. Which drug does *not* potentiate the CNS depression effect of analgesics and hypnotics?

    a. alcohol
    b. antihistamines
    c. corticosteroids
    d. muscle relaxants

31. Which is the most common side effect of prolonged use of haldoperidol (Haldol)?

    a. hypertension
    b. diarrhea
    c. diaphoresis
    d. Parkinsonism

32. Which statement is *not* true of the tricyclic antidepressants?

    a. rapidly effective
    b. causes dry mouth
    c. tranquilizing effect
    d. anticholinergic action

33. Which statement is *not* true of the minor tranquilizers?

    a. for psychosomatic disorders
    b. relieve nausea and vomiting
    c. may cause photosensitivity
    d. useful long term

34. Which statement is *not* true of narcotics?

    a. effects potentiated with antiemetics
    b. treatment for traumatic headaches
    c. can cause hypotension
    d. can cause dependence

35. Which is *not* an appropriate recommendation for someone with an acute back strain?

    a. hot packs
    b. exercise
    c. firm mattress
    d. take aspirin

36. Which medication is used to treat febrile convulsions in children?

    a. Dilantin
    b. Mysoline
    c. Zarontin
    d. Phenobarbital

37. Which is a purpose of the anticonvulsants?

    a. reduce seizures
    b. sedate the patient
    c. cure epilepsy
    d. treat Parkinsonism

38. Which is *not* an antiparkinson drug?

    a. Cimetidine
    b. Cogentin
    c. Sinemet
    d. Symmetrel

39. Which condition is *not* treated with estrogen?

    a. breast engorgement
    b. prostatic cancer
    c. threatened abortion
    d. severe menopausal symptoms

40. Which condition is *not* treated with testosterone?

    a. enuchoidism
    b. androgen deficiency
    c. cryptorchism
    d. metastatic breast cancer
    e. prostate cancer

41. Which is *not* a possible side effect of corticosteroids?

    a. delayed healing
    b. peptic ulcer formation
    c. reduced resistance to infection
    d. hypoglycemia

42. High concentrations of oxygen over prolonged periods of time can cause all of the following *except:*

    a. apnea
    b. acidosis
    c. hiccups
    d. blindness in the newborn

43. The following statements are true of isoproterenol (Isuprel) *except:*

    a. may cause hypoglycemia
    b. may cause palpitations
    c. may be given sublingually
    d. may be used with IPPB

44. The following statements are true of codeine used as an antitussive *except:*

    a. may depress respirations
    b. useful with COPD
    c. may be addictive
    d. classified as narcotic

45. Which of the following stimulates respirations?

    a. Valium
    b. Robaxin
    c. Butazolidin
    d. Carbon dioxide

46. Which is *not* a symptom of hypoglycemia?

    a. tremor
    b. dry skin
    c. irritability
    d. weakness
    e. drowsiness

47. Which is *not* a symptom of hyperglycemia and diabetic acidosis?

    a. nausea and vomiting
    b. fruity breath
    c. labored breathing
    d. sweating
    e. abdominal pain

48. Apical pulse should be taken before giving all of the following drugs *except:*

    a. Inderal
    b. Quinidine
    c. Lanoxin
    d. Nitroglycerin

49. All of the following might be a symptom of digitalis toxicity *except:*

    a. cardiac arrhythmia
    b. blurred vision
    c. urinary retention
    d. GI disturbance

50. Which of the following antihypertensives is *least* likely to cause bradycardia?

    a. Reserpine
    b. Inderal
    c. Apresoline
    d. Catapres

GLOSSARY

Absorption. Passage of a substance through a body surface into body fluids or tissues.

Acetylcholine. Mediator of nerve impulses in the parasympathetic system.

Addiction. Physical and/or psychological dependence on a substance, especially alcohol or drugs, with use of increasing amounts (tolerance) and withdrawal reactions.

Adjunct. Addition to the course of treatment.

Adsorbent. Substance that leads readily to absorption.

Allergic reaction. Response of the body resulting from hypersensitivity to a substance (e.g., rash, hives, and anaphylaxis).

Ampule. Glass container with drug for injection, must be broken at the neck to withdraw drug in solution.

Anaphylaxis. Allergic hypersensitivity reaction of the body to a foreign substance or drug. Mild symptoms include rash, itching, and hives. Severe symptoms include dyspnea, chest constriction, cardiopulmonary collapse, and death.

Angina pectoris. Severe chest pain resulting from decreased blood supply to the heart muscle.

Anorexia. Loss of appetite.

Antagonism. Opposing action of two drugs in which one decreases or cancels out the effect of the other.

Antidote. Substance that neutralizes poisons or toxic substances.

Antineoplastic. Agent that prevents the development, growth, or spreading of malignant cells.

Antipyretic. Medication to reduce fever.

Asymptomatic. No evidence of clinical disease.

Ataxia. Defective muscular coordination, especially with voluntary muscular movements (e.g., walking).

Bactericidal. Destroying bacteria.

Bacteriostatic. Inhibiting or retarding bacterial growth.

Biotransformation. Chemical changes that a substance undergoes in the body.

Bipolar disorder. Manic-depressive mental disorder in which the mood fluctuates from mania to depression.

BPH. Benign prostatic hypertrophy.

Bradycardia. Abnormally slow heartbeat.

Bradykinesia. Abnormally slow movement.

Broad spectrum. Antibiotic effective against a large variety of organisms.

Buccal. In the cheek pouch.

Calculus. Stone.

Cardiotonic. Increasing the force and efficiency of contractions of the heart muscle.

Cardioversion. Correcting an irregular heartbeat (arrhythmia). Usually accomplished by electrical shock (e.g., defibrillation).

Catecholamines. Mediators released at the sympathetic nerve endings (e.g., epinephrine and norepinephrine).

Chemotherapy. Chemicals (drugs) with specific and toxic effects upon disease-producing organisms.

Coenzyme. Enzyme activator.

Concomitant. Taking place at the same time.

Contraindication. Condition or circumstance that indicates that a drug should not be given.

COPD. Chronic obstructive pulmonary disease.

Cryptorchidism. Undescended testicles.

Cumulative effect. Increased effect of a drug that accumulates in the body.

Cycloplegic. Drug that paralyzes the muscles of accommodation for eye examinations.

Cytotoxic. Destroys cells.

Dependence. Acquired need for a drug after repeated use; may be psychological with craving and emotional changes or physical with body changes and withdrawal symptoms.

Drug. Chemical substance taken into the body that affects body function.

Emetic. Agent that induces vomiting.

Endogenous. Produced or originating within a cell or organism.

Endorphin. Endogenous analgesics produced within the body.

Enuresis. Urinary incontinence; bed-wetting.

Enteric coated. Tablet with a special coating that resists disintegration by the gastric juices and desolves in the intestines.

Eunuchism. Lack of male hormone resulting in high-pitched voice and absence of beard and body hair.

Euphoria. Exaggerated feeling of well-being and elation.

Euthyroid. Normal thyroid function.

Excretion. Eliminating waste products of drug metabolism.

Extrapyramidal. Disorder of the brain characterized by tremors, parkinsonlike symptoms, or dystonic twisting of body parts, sometimes associated with prolonged use of antipsychotic drugs.

Flatulence. Excessive gas in the digestive tract.

Generic name. General, common, or nonproprietary name of a drug; begins with lowercase letter.

Glycosuria. Sugar in the urine.

Gout. Form of arthritis in which uric acid crystals are deposited in and around joints.

Homeostasis. Body balance, state of internal equilibrium.

Hypercalcemia. Abnormally high blood calcium.

Hyperglycemia. Abnormally high blood sugar.

Hypersensitivity. Allergic or excessive response of the immune system to a drug or chemical.

Hypoglycemia. Abnormally low blood sugar.

Hypokalemia. Abnormally low blood potassium.

Hypoxia. Deficiency of oxygen.

Idiosyncracy. Unusual reaction to a drug, other than expected.

Immunosuppressive. Decreasing the production of antibodies and phagocytes and depressing the inflammatory reaction.

Indications. List of conditions for which a drug is meant to be used.

Interactions. Actions that occur when two or more drugs are combined, or drugs are combined with certain foods.

Intra-articular (intracapsular). Injected into the joint.

Intradermal (ID). Injected into the layers of the skin.

Intramuscular (IM). Injected into the muscle.

Intravenous (IV). Injected into the vein.

Ischemia. Holding back of the blood; local deficiency of blood supply due to obstruction of circulation to a part (e.g., heart or extremities).

Korsakoff's psychosis. Disorder characterized by polyneuritis, disorientation, mental deterioration, and ataxia with painful foot drop, usually associated with chronic alcoholism.

Legend drug. Available only by prescription.

Local. Affecting one specific area or part.

Lozenge (troche). Tablet that dissolves slowly in the mouth for local effect.

Megadose. Abnormally large dose.

Metabolism. Physical and chemical alterations that a substance undergoes in the body.

Miotic. Drugs that cause the pupil to contract.

Mortar and pestle. Glass cup with glass rod used to crush tablets.

Mydriatic. Drug that dilates the pupil.

Nebulizer (vaporizer). Apparatus for producing a fine spray or mist for inhalation.

Nephrotoxicity. Damage to the kidneys as an adverse reaction to certain drugs.

Objective. Referring to symptoms observed or perceived by others.

Oligospermia. Deficient sperm production.

Ototoxicity. Damage to the eighth nerve resulting in impaired hearing or ringing in the ears (tinnitus); adverse reaction to certain drugs.

Over-the-counter drug (OTC). Medication available without a prescription.

Palliative. Referring to alleviation of symptoms.

Paradoxical. Opposite effect from that expected.

Parenteral. Any route of administration not involving the gastrointestinal tract (e.g., injection, topical, and inhalation).

Photosensitivity. Increased reaction to sunlight with danger of sunburn; adverse reaction to certain drugs.

Placebo. Inactive substance given to simulate the effect of another drug; physical or emotional changes that occur reflect the expectations of the patient.

Placebo effect. Relief from pain as the result of suggestion without active medication.

Potentiation. Increased effect; action of two drugs given simultaneously is greater than the effect of the drugs given separately.

Proliferation. Rapid reproduction.

Prototype. Model or type from which subsequent types arise (e.g., an example of a drug that typifies the characteristics of that classification).

Psychomotor epilepsy. Also known as temporal lobe epilepsy because of the area in the brain that is involved; characterized by temporary impairment of consciousness, confusion, loss of judgment, and abnormal acts, even crimes and hallucinations, but no convulsions.

REM. Rapid eye movement, or dream, phase of sleep.

Selective distribution. Affinity or attraction of a drug to a specific organ or cells.

Status epilepticus. Continual attacks of convulsive seizures without intervals of consciousness.

Subcutaneous (SC). Beneath the skin.

Subjective. Perceived by the individual, not observable by others.

Sublingual (SL). Under the tongue.

Synergism. Action of two drugs working together for increased effect.

Synthetic. Prepared in the laboratory by artificial means.

Systemic. Affecting the whole body or system.

Tachycardia. Abnormally fast heartbeat.

Tardive dyskinesia. Slow, rhythmical, stereotyped, involuntary movements such as tics.

Temporal lobe epilepsy. See *Psychomotor epilepsy.*

Teratogenic effect. Effect of a drug administered to the mother that results in abnormalities in the fetus.

Timed-release capsules (sustained-release or extended-release). Capsules containing many small pellets that are dissolved over a prolonged period of time.

Tinnitus. Ringing in the ears.

Tolerance. Decreased response to a drug after repeated dosage; greater amounts of the drug are required for the same effect.

Topical. Applied to a specific area for a local effect to that area only (e.g., applied to skin or mucous membranes).

Toxicity. Condition resulting from exposure to a poison or a dangerous amount of a drug.

Toxicology. Study and detection of toxic substances, establishing treatment of and methods of prevention of poisoning.

Trade name. Name by which a pharmaceutical company identifies its product; begins with capital letter; brand name.

Transdermal (transcutaneous) delivery system. Patch containing the medicine is applied to the skin; the drug is absorbed through the skin over a prolonged period of time.

Uricosuric. Promoting urinary excretion of uric acid.

Vial. Glass container with rubber stopper that must be punctured with a needle to withdraw a drug solution or to reconstitute a drug in powdered form.

Wernicke's syndrome. Mental disorder characterized by loss of memory, disorientation, and confusion, usually associated with old age or chronic alcoholism.

Withdrawal. Cessation of administration of a drug, especially a narcotic or alcohol, to which a person has become physiologically and/or psychologically addicted; withdrawal symptoms vary with the chemical used.

Index